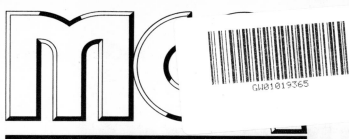

MCQ

For the Higher Examinations

in Clinical
Pharmacology

Gerard McCarthy, FCAnaes, FFARCSI
and
Rajinder Mirakhur, MD, PhD, FFARCS
Department of Anaesthetics, Queen's University of Belfast.

Edward Arnold
A division of Hodder & Stoughton
LONDON MELBOURNE AUCKLAND

©1992 Edward Arnold

First published in Great Britain 1992

British Library Cataloguing in Publication Data

McCarthy, G.
  Multiple Choice Questions in Clinical
  Pharmacology for the Higher Level
  Examination
  I. Title   II. Mirakhur, R. K.
  615

  ISBN 0–340–55792–3

All rights reserved. No part of this publication may be reproduced
or transmitted in any form or by any means, electronically or
mechanically, including photocopying, recording or any
information storage or retrieval system, without either prior
permission in writing from the publisher or a licence permitting
restricted copying. In the United Kingdom such licences are issued
by the Copyright Licensing Agency: 90 Tottenham Court Road,
London W1P 9HE.

Whilst the advice and information in this book is believed to be true
and accurate at the date of going to press, neither the author nor
the publisher can accept any legal responsibility or liability for any
errors or omissions that may be made. In particular (but without
limiting the generality of the preceding disclaimer) every effort has
been made to check drug dosages; however, it is still possible
that errors have been missed. Futhermore, dosage schedules
are constantly being revised and new side-effects recognized.
For these reasons the reader is strongly urged to consult the drug
companies' printed instructions before administering any of the
drugs recommended in this book.

Typeset in Helvetica Light by 'Anneset' Weston-super-Mare, Avon.
Printed and bound in Great Britain for Edward Arnold, a division
of Hodder and Stoughton Limited, Mill Road, Dunton Green,
Sevenoaks, Kent TN13 2YA by R. Clay (St. Ives plc) Bungay,
Suffolk.

Foreword

In their variety of forms, multiple choice questions (MCQs) have become increasingly popular with examiners in pharmacology. When cleverly devised, they are objective and accurate in the assessment that they provide, and allow a detailed coverage of a large proportion of the syllabus. They are valuable, however, not only for examining but for teaching and learning as well. Self assessment by prepared MCQs enables students to structure their learning and to detect their own weaknesses. Furthermore, when the correct answers are given, together with an explanation, as in this case, MCQs become valuable teaching instruments.

The authors of this book are anaesthetists with a special interest in clinical pharmacology. Rajinder Mirakhur is a Senior Lecturer, with long experience of teaching, research and examining for the Fellowship of the Faculty of Anaesthetists in both England and Ireland. Gerard McCarthy is a Postdoctoral Research Fellow in the same department. Together they have devised 300 well-structured, searching questions covering virtually the whole of pharmacology, both pharmacodynamics and pharmacokinetics and some elementary statistics. Students who test themselves against the questions in this book will have reason to be grateful to the authors.

WC Bowman
Glasgow, October 1991

Contents

Introduction

The use of MCQs to test factual recall is now universal as part of higher professional examinations in medicine, as answering MCQs correctly requires a reasonable knowledge and understanding of the subject.

The aim of the book is not only to let the student test what he already knows but also to point out the areas in which his knowledge is lacking. A lot of answers are explained in some detail; however, this book can hardly replace a textbook of pharmacology. For greater depth and understanding the student will always need to consult one of the texts in pharmacology, some of which are listed at the end, and from which many of the answers have been drawn. In the same way not all the drugs in the current pharmacopeia could be discussed here. The emphasis has been on the traditional and the new. Some of the other questions are based on reviews, which could not be listed here in their entirety.

The scope of the questions is wide enough to be useful to postgraduates who have to take an MCQ paper as part of their examination; this includes anaesthetists, pharmacologists and doctors in a wide range of medical specialities. We also hope that it will also be useful to tutors in these disciplines. To get the most out of the book it is advisable that students attempt all the questions in any one section before looking up the answers. Each question, as is usual in examinations, consists of a stem and five statements each of which have to be answered 'true' or 'false'.

We would like to thank Professor WC Bowman for writing the Foreword to the book and to the publishers, Edward Arnold for their help and patience.

Drugs and the cardiovascular system I

1 The Vaughan Williams classification for antiarrhythmic agents:
   (a) Is based on His-bundle recording in patients.
   (b) Has amiodarone as a Class V drug.
   (c) Has verapamil as a Class III drug.
   (d) Has metoprolol as a Class IV drug.
   (e) Has lignocaine as a Class I drug.

2 Lignocaine:
   (a) Blocks fast sodium current activity.
   (b) Prolongs the duration of the action potential.
   (c) Functions best if hypokalaemia is avoided.
   (d) Has a greater negative inotropic effect than disopyramide.
   (e) Acts preferentially on the ischaemic myocardium.

3 Flecainide:
   (a) Has a wider antiarrhythmic spectrum than lignocaine.
   (b) Is a greater negative inotropic agent than lignocaine.
   (c) Must be administered parenterally to produce its therapeutic effect.
   (d) Administration itself can give rise to serious ventricular arrhythmias.
   (e) Exerts no effects on the duration of the QRS complex.

4 Amiodarone:
   (a) Is the only agent to possess Vaughan Williams Class III activity.
   (b) Has minimal negative inotropic effects.
   (c) Has a volume of distribution greater than 3 000 litres in an average adult.
   (d) Has been used successfully in the prophylactic treatment of atrial, junctional and ventricular arrhythmias.
   (e) Therapy is associated with resistance and increased requirements of warfarin.

5 Bretylium:
   (a) Is an adrenergic neurone blocker.
   (b) Is a Vaughan Williams Class V antiarrhythmic.
   (c) Is best given orally.
   (d) Has the major side-effect of hypotension.
   (e) Increases the efficacy of pressor amines.

1 (a) **False** This classification is based on microelectrode studies of the isolated cardiac fibres. The Touboul classification is based on His-bundle recordings.

  (b) **False** There are no Class V drugs according to this classification. Amiodarone is a Class III drug that prolongs the duration of the action potential and the effective refractory period.

  (c) **False** It is a Class IV drug. Commonly known as the calcium entry blockers, this group of drugs inhibits the slow inward calcium-mediated current.

  (d) **False** It is a Class II or beta-adrenoceptor blocking drug.

  (e) **True** These drugs have membrane stabilizing properties.

2 (a) **True** It is a Class I agent.

  (b) **False** Lignocaine is a Class Ib drug and shortens the duration of the action potential. It is Class Ia drugs such as quinidine that may lengthen it.

  (c) **True**

  (d) **False** The negative inotropic effects of disopyramide have been exploited in the treatment of hypertrophic cardiomyopathy.

  (e) **True**

3 (a) **True** But it also possesses more untoward effects.

  (b) **True** This is a commonly encountered adverse effect.

  (c) **False** Flecainide is very well absorbed following oral administration.

  (d) **True** In 8–10 per cent of subjects with malignant ventricular arrhythmias.

  (e) **False** The QRS complex is often markedly widened.

4 (a) **False** It is simply the most important; bretylium, sotalol and N-acetylprocainamide are others.

  (b) **True** It may enhance cardiac performance due to relaxation of vascular smooth muscle and reduction of systemic and coronary vascular resistance.

  (c) **True** It has a large volume of distribution, with an elimination half-life of up to 2 months. It has a long duration of action.

  (d) **True**

  (e) **False** The plasma concentrations of warfarin are increased and its dosage needs to be reduced.

5 (a) **True** It's use is limited to recurrent ventricular fibrillation or ventricular tachycardia where lignocaine and direct current conversion have failed.

  (b) **False** It has Class III activity.

  (c) **False** This drug is only used as an antiarrhythmic in resuscitation and is poorly absorbed orally.

  (d) **True** It inhibits the release of noradrenaline performing a 'chemical sympathectomy'. Although, being a vasodilator, it may rarely improve cardiac output in patients with poor left ventricular function.

  (e) **True**

6 Propafenone:
   (a) Is predominantly a Vaughan Williams Class I antiarrhythmic.
   (b) Is indicated for the treatment of atrial flutter and fibrillation.
   (c) Is of no use in the treatment of ventricular ectopic beats.
   (d) Has negative inotropic effects.
   (e) Is relatively free from extracardiac side-effects.

7 Phenytoin:
   (a) Is a Vaughan Williams Class I antiarrhythmic.
   (b) May be used in the treatment of digitalis-induced arrhythmias.
   (c) May be used to supplement beta-adrenoceptor blockade in cases of pro-
        longed QT syndrome.
   (d) Does not alter the duration of the action potential of atrial tissue.
   (e) May be particularly effective against ventricular arrhythmias after paediatric
        cardiac surgery.

8 Quinidine:
   (a) Increases the duration of the action potential.
   (b) Has no action on atrial arrhythmias.
   (c) Has vagolytic properties.
   (d) Prolongs the QT interval.
   (e) Should be co-prescribed with amiodarone in resistant arrhythmias.

9 Torsades de Pointes:
   (a) May be induced by a combination of sotalol and diuretics.
   (b) May be treated with isoprenaline.
   (c) May be treated with intravenous magnesium sulphate.
   (d) May be treated with amiodarone.
   (e) May be treated with disopyramide.

10 The following drugs are useful for rapid conversion of acute atrial fibrillation to
   sinus rhythm:
   (a) Digoxin.
   (b) Flecainide.
   (c) Sotalol.
   (d) Quinidine.
   (e) Amiodarone.

11 Verapamil:
   (a) Is often associated with rebound hypertension on withdrawal after acute
        intravenous use.
   (b) Has a negative inotropic effect reversible by calcium.
   (c) Exerts its effects on heart rate in man via action at the sinoatrial node.
   (d) Has no effect on platelet aggregation.
   (e) Is antiatherosclerotic.

6 (a) **True**   Although it also shows a very mild beta-adrenoceptor antagonist activity.

    (b) **True**   It is of use in ventricular and supraventricular arrhythmias including the Wolff–Parkinson–White syndrome.

    (c) **False**

    (d) **True**

    (e) **True**   Particularly in comparison with amiodarone.

7 (a) **True**   It is a class Ib drug decreasing the duration of the action potential.

    (b) **True**

    (c) **True**   This is a specific indication for its use.

    (d) **True**

    (e) **True**

8 (a) **True**

    (b) **False**   It has a wide spectrum of activity against ectopic atrial and ventricular activity.

    (c) **True**   This is a feature of the Class Ia agents.

    (d) **True**

    (e) **False**   Quinidine interacts with amiodarone to result in QT prolongation.

9 (a) **True**   This dangerous arrhythmia may require prompt cardioversion with an asynchronous direct current shock.

    (b) **True**   However its use is contraindicated in congenital prolonged QT interval and ischaemic heart disease.

    (c) **True**

    (d) **False**   This would result in a prolongation of the QT interval.

    (e) **False**

10 (a) **False**   This is really the drug of choice for chronic atrial fibrillation. Patients may revert spontaneously because of a general improvement in their condition from treatment.

    (b) **True**   Success rate of over 60 per cent. However, it has a negative inotropic effect and may precipitate heart failure.

    (c) **True**

    (d) **True**   However it has been superseded by drugs such as amiodarone and flecainide.

    (e) **True**   Furthermore this drug is not as negative an inotrope as flecainide. The treatment of choice for acute conversion is cardioversion. Drugs have a place only if the patient is unsuitable or for prevention of relapse.

11 (a) **False**   Highly unlikely.

    (b) **True**

    (c) **False**   Verapamil decreases the rate of phase-4 spontaneous depolarization in cardiac Purkinje fibres, blocking the delayed after-depolarizations and triggered activity.

    (d) **False**   Verapamil inhibits human platelet aggregation.

    (e) **True**

12 Calcium chloride:
  (a) Shortens ventricular systole.
  (b) Increases the duration of the effective refractory period.
  (c) Provides protection against ischaemic brain damage.
  (d) May be used to treat cardiac depression following massive infusions of citrated blood.
  (e) Improves survival in cardiac asystole.

13 Verapamil:
  (a) Is useful in the treatment of the arrhythmias of digoxin toxicity.
  (b) Bioavailability increases with prolonged oral administration.
  (c) May be usefully combined with prazosin.
  (d) Is the agent of choice in controlling the tachycardia associated with the sick sinus syndrome.
  (e) And disopyramide are an ideal combination for the treatment of cardiac arrhythmias.

14 Diltiazem:
  (a) Is a more potent vasodilator than verapamil.
  (b) Has a greater negative chronotropic effect than nifedipine.
  (c) Is free from effects on the atrioventricular node.
  (d) Has a greater negative inotropic effect than verapamil.
  (e) Is superior to other calcium channel blockers in the treatment of coronary artery spasm.

15 Use of calcium channel blockers may be associated with:
  (a) Diarrhoea.
  (b) Peripheral oedema.
  (c) Rebound increase in angina on sudden withdrawal of treatment.
  (d) Flushing.
  (e) Bronchospasm.

16 Nifedipine:
  (a) May precipitate congestive heart failure.
  (b) May occasionally precipitate myocardial ischaemia.
  (c) As opposed to nitrates suffers from the disadvantage of a shorter duration of action.
  (d) Is a more potent coronary vasodilator than the nitrates.
  (e) Has a more potent effect on arterioles than the nitrates.

12 (a) **True**   High serum calcium concentrations shorten ventricular systole and also decrease the duration of the effective refractory period.
   (b) **False**
   (c) **False**
   (d) **True**
   (e) **False**   Calcium does not increase survival in asystole. Its use in conditions of myocardial ischaemia may lead to an increase in infarct size.

13 (a) **False**   Verapamil, particularly by the intravenous route, is contraindicated in the treatment of digoxin toxicity because of the danger of increasing atrioventricular block. In addition – it decreases the renal clearance of digoxin.
   (b) **True**   Because of saturation of hepatic metabolism.
   (c) **True**   The two drugs seem to be synergistic in producing peripheral vasodilatation.
   (d) **False**   It is contraindicated in this condition.
   (e) **False**   Because of the combined negative inotropic effects of the two drugs.

14 (a) **False**
   (b) **True**   Nifedipine does not influence the sinoatrial node or the atrioventricular node; if anything, it may cause a reflex increase in heart rate.
   (c) **False**   It slows atrioventricular conduction like verapamil.
   (d) **False**   Verapamil is more cardiodepressant.
   (e) **False**   All the drugs are similar in this respect.

15 (a) **False**   Constipation is the usual side-effect.
   (b) **True**   As a consequence of their vasodilator properties.
   (c) **True**
   (d) **True**
   (e) **False**   An advantage of these drugs over beta-adrenergic receptor blocking agents is freedom from bronchoconstriction. There may actually be a beneficial effect from the prevention of bronchoconstriction.

16 (a) **True**   Because of negative inotropic effects, particularly if myocardial function is poor.
   (b) **True**   This may be a 'steal' phenomenon in a small number of cases.
   (c) **False**   Calcium antagonists differ from the nitrates in not only being more potent but also having a more sustained action.
   (d) **True**
   (e) **True**

17 Verapamil:
   (a) Induces less cardiovascular depression during anaesthesia with enflurane than with isoflurane.
   (b) May interact with halothane to increase the risk of heart block.
   (c) Is of no value in obtunding the haemodynamic response to tracheal intubation in anaesthetized patients.
   (d) Reduces the MAC of halothane.
   (e) May potentiate a vecuronium-induced neuromuscular blockade.

18 Verapamil:
   (a) And theophylline show a significant interaction.
   (b) Interacts with digoxin by increasing its renal tubular secretion.
   (c) Interacts with carbamazepine by increasing its steady state plasma levels.
   (d) And cyclosporin show no significant interaction.
   (e) Administration results in a decreased quinidine clearance.

19 Enoximone:
   (a) Raises arterial pressure at the expense of splanchnic and renal vasoconstriction.
   (b) May induce hypotension.
   (c) Is a direct cardiac beta-adrenoceptor stimulant.
   (d) Causes an increase in activator calcium in the myocardium.
   (e) May lead to bronchoconstriction.

20 Enoximone:
   (a) Is effective only when given intravenously.
   (b) Is the inotrope of choice in renal failure.
   (c) Is a pulmonary artery vasodilator.
   (d) Is beneficial when used simultaneously with dobutamine in low output states.
   (e) Must be administered in 5 per cent dextrose.

21 Noradrenaline:
   (a) Is a pure alpha-adrenoceptor agonist.
   (b) Has potent bronchodilator activity.
   (c) Increases myocardial oxygen consumption.
   (d) Increases skeletal muscle blood flow.
   (e) Elevates pulmonary capillary wedge pressure.

17 (a) **False** It is more during enflurane anaesthesia.
   (b) **True**
   (c) **False** Verapamil does obtund the hypertensive response. It has a hypotensive effect on acute administration although the effect is transient.
   (d) **True**
   (e) **True** This has, however been shown mostly in *in vitro* studies. While there are a couple of case reports about difficulty in antagonising neuromuscular blockade in humans, there is not a great deal of published evidence in humans to support this.

18 (a) **True** The plasma concentrations of theophylline are increased.
   (b) **False** The steady state serum digoxin concentration is elevated.
   (c) **True** The steady state plasma concentrations of carbamazepine increases by about 50 per cent.
   (d) **False** The cyclosporin plasma levels are raised by inhibition of hepatic metabolism.
   (e) **True** Verapamil decreases quinidine clearance by 50 per cent.

19 (a) **False**
   (b) **True** Enoximone has vasodilating properties, which will lead to hypotension if the preload is inadequate.
   (c) **False** It is a selective phosphodiesterase inhibitor.
   (d) **True** Inhibition of phosphodiesterases results in accumulation of cyclic-AMP, which in turn leads to the phosphorylation of protein kinases. This results in slow calcium channels remaining open for longer, hence more calcium accumulates in the sarcoplasmic reticulum, which is released during depolarization, therefore enhancing contractility.
   (e) **False** Although primarily a vasodilator and inotrope, enoximone has a bronchodilating effect. In addition, it increases diaphragmatic muscle contraction.

20 (a) **False** It can be given orally.
   (b) **False** Although subject to hepatic metabolism, it has an active metabolite piroximone that is dependent on renal excretion.
   (c) **True**
   (d) **True** This is a useful interaction.
   (e) **False** It may crystallize in 5 per cent dextrose; water or normal saline is suitable.

21 (a) **False** It also has weak beta$_1$-adrenoceptor activity.
   (b) **False** It has no bronchodilator action.
   (c) **True**
   (d) **False** Its alpha-adrenoceptor effects are dominant.
   (e) **True**

22 Dopexamine:
   (a) Is a selective phosphodiesterase inhibitor.
   (b) Produces splanchnic and renal vasoconstriction.
   (c) May be given orally.
   (d) Tends to increase the pulmonary capillary wedge pressure.
   (e) Has a similar arrthymogenic potential to dopamine.

23 Dobutamine:
   (a) Is a less potent inotropic agent than isoprenaline.
   (b) Is more likely to result in a decrease in peripheral vascular resistance than dopamine.
   (c) Causes a reduction in pulmonary capillary wedge pressure.
   (d) Is a more potent $beta_1$-adrenoceptor agonist than dopamine.
   (e) Is active at D_1 but not D_2 receptors.

24 Dopexamine:
   (a) Is a less potent $beta_1$-adrenergic receptor agonist than dopamine.
   (b) Is primarily active at D_2 receptors.
   (c) Shows no alpha-adrenoceptor activity.
   (d) Is a more potent renal vasodilator than dopamine.
   (e) Unlike dopamine, does not induce nausea.

25 Digoxin:
   (a) Shortens the PR interval.
   (b) Flattens the ST segment.
   (c) Causes peaking of the T wave.
   (d) Shortens the QT interval.
   (e) Increases the resting membrane potential.

26 Digoxin toxicity is commonly manifested as:
   (a) Muscular hyperexcitability.
   (b) Visual aberrations.
   (c) Psychosis.
   (d) Premature ventricular ectopic beats.
   (e) Atrioventricular junctional tachycardia.

27 Digoxin toxicity is likely in the presence of:
   (a) Hyperkalaemia.
   (b) Hypomagnesaemia.
   (c) Amiodarone.
   (d) Hyperthyroidism.
   (e) Hypercalcaemia.

22 (a) **False**   Dopexamine is a catecholamine with $beta_2$-adrenergic receptor agonist properties and the ability to inhibit noradrenaline re-uptake.
  (b) **False**   Dopexamine produces splanchnic and renal vasodilatation.
  (c) **False**
  (d) **False**   Dopexamine tends to reduce the pulmonary capillary wedge pressure slightly.
  (e) **False**   Dopexamine tends to have a lower incidence of arrhythmias.

23 (a) **False**   It is more potent although it is a synthetic derivative of isoprenaline.
  (b) **True**   Because of its primary $beta_1$-receptor stimulant action.
  (c) **True**
  (d) **True**
  (e) **False**   It is not active at either receptor.

24 (a) **True**   Dopexamine does not show $beta_1$-receptor stimulant properties at clinically used doses. However, it has potent $beta_2$-receptor agonist properties.
  (b) **False**   Dopexamine has greater activity at D_1 receptors.
  (c) **True**
  (d) **False**   Renal vasodilatation is a D_1 receptor property; dopexamine is only about a third as potent as dopamine in this respect.
  (e) **False**   Nausea is a D_2 property, both drugs are active on these receptors in the chemoreceptor trigger zone.

25 (a) **False**   The ECG effects of digoxin include prolongation of the PR interval, flattening of the ST segment, depression of the T wave and shortening of the QT interval. Digoxin inhibits the membrane-bound Na^+/K^+ ATPase pump so that intracellular sodium levels rise, which leads to an increased intracellular calcium level.
  (b) **True**
  (c) **False**
  (d) **True**
  (e) **False**

26 (a) **False**   It causes fatigue.
  (b) **True**
  (c) **False**   It is uncommon although other types of central nervous system disturbances do occur.
  (d) **True**
  (e) **True**

27 (a) **False**   It is common in the presence of hypokalaemia.
  (b) **True**
  (c) **True**
  (d) **False**
  (e) **True**

28 Milrinone:
   (a) Is a Na+/K+ ATPase inhibitor.
   (b) Is an inotrope whose use is limited by vasoconstriction.
   (c) Causes an appreciable increase in myocardial oxygen consumption.
   (d) Use may be complicated by thrombocytopenia.
   (e) Shows no inotropic effect in a fully digitalized patient.

29 Xamoterol:
   (a) Is a new synthetic cardiac glycoside.
   (b) Is indicated in the treatment of severe congestive heart failure.
   (c) Has no vasodilating effect.
   (d) Does not usually cause an increase in heart rate.
   (e) Has therapeutically beneficial bronchodilating effects.

30 Digoxin is contraindicated in:
   (a) The treatment of congestive heart failure in the presence of atrial fibrillation.
   (b) Heart failure in acute myocardial infarction.
   (c) The Wolff-Parkinson-White syndrome.
   (d) Hypertrophic obstructive cardiomyopathy.
   (e) In children with high output states due to left to right shunts.

31 Methoxamine:
   (a) Is not metabolized by monoamine oxidase.
   (b) Increases cardiac output by a direct action.
   (c) Does not cause cerebral stimulation.
   (d) Is useful in the treatment of paroxysmal atrial tachycardia.
   (e) Is more likely to show tachyphylaxis than ephedrine.

32 Phenylephrine:
   (a) Is predominantly a direct beta-adrenoceptor agonist.
   (b) Causes miosis while ephedrine causes mydriasis.
   (c) Increases the cardiac output.
   (d) Should not be used to treat hypotension due to spinal or epidural anaesthesia in labour.
   (e) Decreases the renal blood flow while increasing the arterial pressure.

33 Metaraminol:
   (a) Has both alpha- and beta-adrenoceptor agonist effects.
   (b) Has a sedative effect.
   (c) Should preferably be avoided during halothane anaesthesia.
   (d) Is useful in the treatment of anorexia.
   (e) Is the safest vasopressor to use in the presence of monoamine oxidase inhibitors.

34 Isoprenaline:
   (a) Unlike noradrenaline results in an increase in cardiac output in normal individuals.
   (b) Like methoxamine results in reflex bradycardia.
   (c) Unlike adrenaline has no effect on histamine release.
   (d) Unlike sotalol is useful in the treatment of Torsades de Pointes.
   (e) Unlike adrenaline results in hypoglycaemia.

28 (a) **False** Milrinone is a selective inhibitor of peak III phosphodiesterase isoenzyme in cardiac muscle (incidently it is about 20 times more potent than amrinone in this respect).
   (b) **False** It is a vasodilator.
   (c) **False**
   (d) **True**
   (e) **False**

29 (a) **False** Xamoterol is a beta$_1$-adrenoceptor blocking drug with high intrinsic sympathomimetic activity.
   (b) **False** The indications for xamoterol are now being reduced in number.
   (c) **True**
   (d) **True** Because of its beta-adrenoceptor blocking properties.
   (e) **False** (see (a) above).

30 (a) **False** Congestive cardiac failure and atrial fibrillation are both indications for digoxin.
   (b) **True** It is a relative contraindication because of the risk of increasing the infarct size and provoking arrhythmias.
   (c) **True**
   (d) **True** It is a contraindication.
   (e) **False** It is generally useful and preferable to diuretics.

31 (a) **True** Nor is it inactivated by COMT, hence its long duration of action.
   (b) **False** It is a vasoconstrictor.
   (c) **True** This is a feature of ephedrine.
   (d) **True**
   (e) **False** Tachyphylaxis is more a feature of ephedrine.

32 (a) **False** Phenylephrine is a potent direct alpha-adrenoceptor agonist.
   (b) **False** Both cause mydriasis.
   (c) **False** It is generally unchanged or reduced.
   (d) **True** Potent alpha-adrenergic receptor stimulants result in a decrease in uterine blood flow.
   (e) **True**

33 (a) **True** In addition it has both direct and indirect effects.
   (b) **False**
   (c) **True** Due to the possibility of arrhythmias.
   (d) **False**
   (e) **False** Due to the possibility of interaction leading to severe hypertension.

34 (a) **True** Because of an increase in both the heart rate and the cardiac contractility. Noradrenaline on the other hand, results in vasoconstriction and a reflex bradycardia that tends to limit any rise in cardiac output.
   (b) **False** Isoprenaline is useful in the treatment of low heart rates and heart block.
   (c) **False** Both inhibit histamine liberation.
   (d) **True**
   (e) **False** Although isoprenaline causes less marked hyperglycaemia.

35 Dopamine:
  (a) Induced renal vasodilatation is antagonised by propranolol.
  (b) In doses of 2–5 μg/kg/minute results in marked increase in peripheral resistance.
  (c) Depletes presynaptic stores of noradrenaline.
  (d) Gives rise to arrhythmias more often than dobutamine.
  (e) Is as potent a beta$_2$-receptor agonist as dopexamine.

Drugs and the cardiovascular system II

36 Beta-adrenoceptor blocking agents:
  (a) Benefit the ischaemic myocardium if the preload rises substantially in the course of the therapy.
  (b) Benefit the myocardium in all types of angina.
  (c) Are of value in Raynaud's disease.
  (d) Are of value in migraine.
  (e) Should not be used in the acute treatment of Wolff-Parkinson-White syndrome.

37 In myocardial ischaemia, beta-adrenoceptor blockade:
  (a) Decreases the risk of ventricular fibrillation.
  (b) Decreases the size of the infarct due to coronary occlusion.
  (c) By agents with high intrinsic sympathomimetic activity decreases the risk of reinfarction.
  (d) If withdrawn, leads abruptly to an increased risk of infarction.
  (e) Decreases the incidence of arrhythmias associated with intubation.

38 Treatment with beta-adrenoceptor blocking drugs:
  (a) Decreases the hypermetabolic state of thyrotoxicosis.
  (b) Has no influence on the vascularity of a hyperactive thyroid gland.
  (c) With intrinsic sympathomimetic activity is useful during a thyroid storm.
  (d) Controls the tremor of thyrotoxicosis.
  (e) Paradoxically raises free thyroxine levels.

39 Cardioselectivity in beta-adrenoceptor blocking agents:
  (a) Is well maintained only at relatively low doses.
  (b) Makes these drugs more effective anti-anginal agents than non-selective drugs.
  (c) Limits their usefulness in the treatment of migraine.
  (d) Is of special value in the patient with glaucoma.
  (e) Is not related to their antihypertensive activity.

40 Sotalol:
  (a) Is useful in the treatment of QT interval prolongation.
  (b) Is useful in hypertension with symptomatic arrhythmias.
  (c) Possesses Class I and Class IV effects according to Vaughan Williams classification.
  (d) Is contraindicated during treatment with amiodarone.
  (e) Administration is contraindicated in Torsades de Pointes.

41 Prazosin:
  (a) Is a presynaptic alpha$_2$-receptor agonist.
  (b) Is limited in usefulness by troublesome tachycardia.
  (c) Therapy may be associated with both tachyphylaxis and tolerance.
  (d) May produce urinary retention.
  (e) Should not be used in patients with severe congestive cardiac failure.

35 (a) **False** It may be partly antagonized by butyrophenones.
   (b) **False** This effect is seen at much higher doses.
   (c) **True** This can become a limiting factor in its use because of the partial indirect effects of the drug.
   (d) **True**
   (e) **False** Dopexamine is much more potent in this respect.

---

36 (a) **False** These drugs may induce heart failure.
   (b) **False** Beta-receptor blockade is not useful in Prinzmetal's variant angina because of unopposed alpha-receptor activity.
   (c) **False**
   (d) **True** The effect is prophylactic and seems limited to agents without intrinsic sympathomimetic activity.
   (e) **True**

37 (a) **True**
   (b) **True** By up to 30 per cent.
   (c) **False** The risk of reinfarction and sudden death are reduced but this benefit may be limited to drugs without intrinsic sympathomimetic activity.
   (d) **True**
   (e) **True**

38 (a) **False** The benefits of this therapy are symptomatic and not due to control of the hypermetabolic state.
   (b) **True**
   (c) **False** These patients have increased sympathomimetic activity.
   (d) **True** Because of its sympathomimetic basis.
   (e) **False**

39 (a) **True** It may be lost when they are used in high doses.
   (b) **False** All such drugs appear to be equally effective.
   (c) **False** Intrinsic sympathomimetic activity and not the cardioselectivity is the important factor in the therapy of migraine with these agents.
   (d) **False**
   (e) **True**

40 (a) **False** Most beta-receptor blocking agents with the exception of sotalol are used for this condition as it may itself prolong the QT interval.
   (b) **True**
   (c) **False** It has Class II and Class III effects.
   (d) **True** Sotalol should not be given with agents which prolong the QT interval.
   (e) **True** Sotalol may give rise to this state.

41 (a) **False** It is a postsynaptic alpha$_1$-receptor blocking drug.
   (b) **False** Although a vasodilator, excessive tachycardia is rarely a problem with prazosin. Hypotension following the start of therapy on the other hand, can be a problem.
   (c) **True**
   (d) **False** It is marketed as a treatment for retention.
   (e) **False** Prazosin is useful because of its ability to reduce arteriolar resistance and increase venous pooling.

42 Phenoxybenzamine:
   (a) Is a non-competitive alpha-adrenergic antagonist.
   (b) Is of therapeutic value in benign prostatic obstruction.
   (c) Inhibits the release of noradrenaline from adrenergic nerves.
   (d) Can be used as a nasal decongestant.
   (e) Produces a reduction in arterial pressure by reduction of peripheral resistance and cardiac output.

43 Phentolamine:
   (a) Is a specific competitive alpha$_1$-adrenergic antagonist.
   (b) Acts within minutes of administration.
   (c) Is contraindicated in the presence of monoamine oxidase inhibitors.
   (d) Unlike phenoxybenzamine does not cause reflex tachycardia.
   (e) Does not have negative inotropic effects.

44 Guanethidine:
   (a) Has a reserpine-like action.
   (b) Can be used intravenously for rapid control of hypertension in phaeochromocytoma.
   (c) Is useful in the treatment of causalgia.
   (d) Administration may be complicated by constipation.
   (e) Administration may result in oedema.

45 Trimetaphan:
   (a) Is a postsynaptic alpha$_1$-adrenergic antagonist.
   (b) Has a rapid onset of effect.
   (c) Is primarily a smooth muscle relaxant.
   (d) Is metabolized by acetylcholinesterase and may thus affect the duration of action of suxamethonium.
   (e) Often causes dilated pupils.

46 Clonidine:
   (a) Is a presynaptic alpha$_2$-adrenoceptor blocking agent.
   (b) Has relatively little effect on peripheral resistance.
   (c) May frequently cause postural hypotension.
   (d) Therapy is complicated by reflex tachycardia.
   (e) May be useful in the treatment of opiate addiction.

47 Clonidine:
   (a) Exhibits analgesic properties on extradural administration.
   (b) Exhibits analgesic properties on transdermal administration.
   (c) Therapy is complicated by mouth dryness.
   (d) Administration on a chronic basis may result in diarrhoea.
   (e) Withdrawal does not cause rebound hypertension unless treatment has been continued for more than 4 weeks.

42 (a) **True**   It binds covalently to the receptors.

   (b) **True**   Because of action on the alpha-receptors at the base of the bladder.

   (c) **False**   The release of noradrenaline is actually increased because of $alpha_2$-blockade resulting in tachycardia.

   (d) **False**   It may produce nasal congestion.

   (e) **False**   While the peripheral resistance is decreased, the cardiac output may actually be increased.

43 (a) **False**   Non-specific competitive $alpha_1$- and $alpha_2$-adrenergic antagonist.

   (b) **True**

   (c) **False**   It is useful in the treatment of hypertensive reactions due to monoamine oxidase inhibition.

   (d) **False**   The two are similar in this respect.

   (e) **True**

44 (a) **True**   Although it is primarily a ganglion blocking drug.

   (b) **False**   It is contraindicated as it may provoke a marked hypertensive response.

   (c) **True**   It is used in the treatment of sympathetic dystrophy (causalgia) by intravenous regional administration.

   (d) **False**   It results in diarrhoea due to unopposed parasympathetic activity.

   (e) **True**   Hence to be avoided in congestive heart failure.

45 (a) **False**   It is a ganglion blocking agent.

   (b) **True**   But tachyphylaxis may result.

   (c) **False**   (See (a) above). It may also show some direct myocardial depressant effect.

   (d) **False**   It is metabolized by plasma cholinesterase and may also be an inhibitor of this enzyme, that is the reason for the prolongation of the effect of suxamethonium.

   (e) **True**

46 (a) **False**   It is an $alpha_2$-agonist, postsynaptic in the central nervous system but presynaptic in the periphery. Stimulation of these receptors appears to inhibit the outflow from the vasomotor centre. Its use may be associated with bradycardia.

   (b) **True**

   (c) **False**   It is rare as homeostatic reflexes tend to be preserved.

   (d) **False**   (See (c) above).

   (e) **True**

47 (a) **True**

   (b) **True**

   (c) **True**   Due to inhibition of cholinergic transmission to the salivary glands.

   (d) **False**   Constipation can be a problem with clonidine administration.

   (e) **False**   This can occur after treatment periods of as little as 7 days.

48 Methyldopa:
  (a) Is metabolized to methylnoradrenaline in the central nervous system for exerting its antihypertensive effect.
  (b) Is a directly acting vasodilator.
  (c) Is useful in the treatment of phaeochromocytoma.
  (d) Administration may be complicated by sedation.
  (e) Has the advantage of not causing postural hypotension.

49 In the eye:
  (a) Phenyleprine is a miotic.
  (b) Cyclopentolate is a mydriatic.
  (c) Pilocarpine is a miotic.
  (d) Ecothiopate is a mydriatic.
  (e) Timolol is a miotic.

50 Sodium nitroprusside:
  (a) Produces nitric oxide, which results in vasodilatation.
  (b) relaxes arteriolar smooth muscle selectively.
  (c) Should not be administered at a rate greater than 8 μg/kg/minute.
  (d) May cause an increase in intracranial pressure.
  (e) Has no effect on bleeding time.

51 Sodium nitroprusside:
  (a) Administration results in an increase in pulmonary artery pressure in patients with cardiac failure.
  (b) Decreases plasma renin activity.
  (c) Administration results in less tachycardia than diazoxide.
  (d) Increases intrapulmonary shunting.
  (e) Toxicity is characterized by metabolic acidosis without an increase in plasma lactate concentrations.

52 Nitroglycerine:
  (a) Is contraindicated in hypertrophic obstructive cardiomyopathy.
  (b) Is predominantly an arteriolar dilator.
  (c) Unlike nitroprusside raises intracranial pressure.
  (d) Is ideally administered from rigid polyvinyl chloride containers as it is incompatible with polyethylene.
  (e) Is less likely than nitroprusside to lead to rebound hypertension.

53 Diazoxide:
  (a) Has diuretic activity.
  (b) Is associated with hyperglycaemia.
  (c) Is a potent uterine relaxant.
  (d) Is not usually associated with tachycardia because of its weak beta-adrenergic blocking action.
  (e) Increases the coronary blood flow.

48 (a) **True**
   (b) **False**   It acts centrally by stimulating alpha$_2$-adrenergic receptors.
   (c) **False**
   (d) **True**
   (e) **False**

49 (a) **False**   It is a sympathetic stimulant.
   (b) **True**   A useful anticholinergic drug with a short duration of action.
   (c) **True**   Hence useful in the treatment of glaucoma.
   (d) **False**   An irreversible anticholinesterase with miotic activity.
   (e) **False**   It has little effect on the size of the pupil.

50 (a) **True**   Nitric oxide produced from nitroprusside activates guanylate
                   cyclase which increases the cyclic-GMP production activating
                   the cyclic-GMP-dependent protein kinase and eventually dephos-
                   phorylation of myosin light chains producing smooth muscle
                   relaxation.
   (b) **False**   It relaxes both arterial and venous smooth muscle.
   (c) **True**   Otherwise toxicity may result.
   (d) **True**   Sometimes without an increase in cerebral blood flow.
   (e) **False**   It produces a dose-dependent increase in bleeding time.

51 (a) **False**   It is reduced.
   (b) **False**   It is increased and may be the reason for rebound hypertension on
                   withdrawal of the drug.
   (c) **True**
   (d) **True**   With the risk of hypoxia.
   (e) **False**   Lactic acidosis results during toxicity because of histotoxic anoxia.

52 (a) **True**
   (b) **False**   It acts predominantly on capacitance vessels.
   (c) **False**   They both raise intracranial pressure.
   (d) **False**   It is the other way round.
   (e) **True**   It is slower in both onset and offset, and has minimal effects on the
                   renin–angiotensin system.

53 (a) **False**   Although it is related to chlorothiazide it lacks the sulphonamide
                   group.
   (b) **True**   By blocking insulin release. This may be useful in cases of islet cell
                   neoplasia.
   (c) **True**
   (d) **False**   It causes tachycardia and has no beta-adrenergic blocking action.
   (e) **True**

54 Hydralazine:
  (a) Toxicity is more likely in fast acetylators due to formation of the acetylated metabolite.
  (b) Although a vasodilator acts predominantly by an alpha-adrenoceptor blocking action.
  (c) Therapy is complicated by severe postural hypotension.
  (d) May lead to peripheral neuropathy.
  (e) Administration is associated with increased renin activity.

55 Hypotension induced by adenosine:
  (a) Is due to a reduction in cardiac output.
  (b) Is associated with a compensatory tachycardia.
  (c) Is rapid in onset.
  (d) Is accompanied by uric acid accumulation.
  (e) Is potentiated by dipyridamole.

56 Minoxidil:
  (a) Should usually not be administered without concurrent therapy with a diuretic.
  (b) Is a selective dilator of capacitance vessels.
  (c) Administration may result in alopecia.
  (d) Is preferably given along with a beta-adrenoceptor blocking drug.
  (e) Is useful for its uricosuric effect.

57 Ketanserin:
  (a) Is a serotonin agonist.
  (b) Has useful alpha-adrenoceptor antagonist properties.
  (c) Increases blood viscosity.
  (d) Is useful in the intraoperative management of the carcinoid syndrome.
  (e) Is a useful treatment for congenital prolonged QT interval.

58 Doxazosin:
  (a) Is a directly acting vasodilator.
  (b) Has the disadvantage of causing postural hypotension.
  (c) Is frequently associated with 'first-dose' hypotension within an hour of administration.
  (d) Pharmacokinetics are not altered in impaired renal function.
  (e) Is not associated with a rise in low-density lipoproteins.

54 (a) **False** It is the slow acetylators who are more likely to show toxicity. Moreover it is either the drug itself or its non-acetylated metabolite that are probably responsible.
   (b) **False** Although the drug has this effect it acts predominantly as an arteriolar dilator.
   (c) **False** Because of the preferential dilatation of the arterioles.
   (d) **True** By producing pyridoxine deficiency.
   (e) **True** As a result of increased sympathetic activity. Fluid retention and congestive cardiac failure may thus occur.

55 (a) **False** It is a vasodilator.
   (b) **False** The changes in heart rate are minimal.
   (c) **True** In addition has a very short plasma half-life.
   (d) **False** This was a feature of adenosine triphosphate (ATP).
   (e) **True** Because dipyridamole is an adenosine uptake inhibitor.

56 (a) **True** It is very prone to causing fluid retention.
   (b) **False** It is an almost pure arteriolar dilator.
   (c) **False** It leads to hypertrichosis possibly due to increased cutaneous blood flow.
   (d) **True** (See (b) above).
   (e) **False** It may cause hyperuricaemia and hyperglycaemia.

57 (a) **False** It is a serotonin (5-HT$_2$) antagonist. Vascular endothelium has both 5-HT$_1$ and 5-HT$_2$ receptors, the former mediate vasodilatation and are probably found predominantly in arterioles, the latter mediate vasoconstriction and are found in the larger arteries. The inhibition of 5-HT$_2$ receptors seems to potentiate the action of 5-HT$_1$ receptors. For these reasons ketanserin is being evaluated as treatment in chronic leg ulcers, intermittent claudication and Raynaud's disease.
   (b) **True** It can be used as an antihypertensive agent with roughly equivalent efficacy as metoprolol. The exact mode of action is unclear and the drug may act both as an alpha-adrenoceptor and as a 5-HT antagonist.
   (c) **False** It may decrease whole blood viscosity possibly by haemodilution or an increase in the red cell deformability. It also decreases 5-HT-induced platelet aggregation.
   (d) **True** It is very effective in controlling the hypertensive responses in patients with the carcinoid syndrome.
   (e) **False** Prolonged QT interval of any type is a contraindication for its use. Ketanserin is particularly liable to prolong the QT interval in the presence of hypokalaemia and bradycardia with an increased risk of arrhythmias.

58 (a) **False** It is a postjunctional alpha$_1$-adrenergic antagonist notable for freedom from reflex tachycardia.
   (b) **True** It is the main side-effect of this drug and is a typical vasodilator effect.
   (c) **False** On both counts. Maximum effect takes about 2–6hours.
   (d) **True**
   (e) **True** Unlike the beta-adrenoceptor blocking drugs it actually improves the plasma lipid profile.

59 Esmolol:
   (a) Is cardioselective in its effects.
   (b) Has significant intrinsic sympathomimetic activity.
   (c) Has no active metabolites.
   (d) Shows a prolonged duration of action in those with atypical plasma cholinesterases.
   (e) Treatment should be limited to 2 hours due to the risk of methanol intoxication.

60 Enalapril:
   (a) Depends upon hepatic metabolism for its therapeutic effect.
   (b) Is shorter acting than captopril.
   (c) Is half as potent as captopril.
   (d) Decreases renal vascular resistance without changing glomerular filtration.
   (e) May be associated with unpredictable hypotension during or after anaesthesia and surgery.

61 Captopril:
   (a) Has no influence on the dose requirement of sodium nitroprusside- induced hypotension.
   (b) Is ineffective in hypertension with a high-renin state.
   (c) Induces glucose intolerance.
   (d) Is a mixed vasodilator.
   (e) Should not be co-prescribed with indomethacin.

62 Captopril:
   (a) May induce proteinuria.
   (b) Has the same incidence of neutropenia as enalapril.
   (c) Is useful in diabetics as its slows the progression of nephropathy.
   (d) Is ineffective in normotensive subjects.
   (e) Unlike enalapril, is free from the risk of angioedema.

63 Quinapril:
   (a) Frequently causes hyponatraemia.
   (b) Results in raised catecholamine levels.
   (c) Results in raised aldosterone levels.
   (d) Frequently results in impotence.
   (e) May result in a chronic cough.

64 Sodium reabsorption following filtration in the glomerulus is reduced by about:
   (a) 20 per cent by bendrofluazide.
   (b) 5 per cent by amiloride.
   (c) 2 per cent by acetazolamide.
   (d) 60 per cent by frusemide.
   (e) 20 per cent by mannitol.

59 (a) **True**   And in addition it is short acting.
   (b) **False**   Its intrinsic sympathomimetic activity is minimal.
   (c) **True**
   (d) **False**   It is metabolized by red blood cell esterases, and hence its duration of action is unaffected in those with atypical plasma cholinesterases.
   (e) **False**   It is true that one of the metabolites of esmolol is methanol but the quantities liberated are insignificant; the major limiting factor in treatment is hypotension.

60 (a) **True**   As it is a prodrug that needs to be hydrolysed to the active agent enalaprilat.
   (b) **False**   It is the longer acting of the two. Most angiotensin converting enzyme (ACE) inhibitor drugs on the market are long acting. The shorter acting drugs may have a marginal advantage in heart failure.
   (c) **False**   Enalapril is about twice as potent.
   (d) **True**
   (e) **True**   ACE inhibitors are also well known to be associated with unpredictable hypotension on first administration especially in the hypovolaemic.

61 (a) **False**   The dose requirements of the latter are reduced.
   (b) **False**   It is most effective in high-renin states but still shows activity even in low-renin states.
   (c) **False**   ACE inhibitors are free from adverse effects on glucose, uric acid and cholesterol metabolism.
   (d) **True**   It is both an arterial dilator and a venodilator.
   (e) **True**   Indomethacin attenuates the effects of captopril.

62 (a) **True**   Especially in high doses.
   (b) **False**   Captopril has a higher incidence of neutropenia due to its effects on the bone marrow.
   (c) **True**   Even though such drugs may induce proteinuria.
   (d) **False**   It lowers the arterial pressure in both hypertensive and normotensive subjects.
   (e) **False**

63 (a) **False**
   (b) **False**   Angiotensin II is required for the normal release of noradrenaline.
   (c) **False**   It lowers the aldosterone levels.
   (d) **False**   ACE inhibitors are noted for their lack of adverse effects on the quality of life.
   (e) **True**   The mechanism is not clear, but may involve bradykinin and pulmonary receptors.

64 (a) **False**   The maximum is about 10 per cent.
   (b) **True**
   (c) **True**
   (d) **False**   The maximum amount is only 35–40 per cent.
   (e) **False**   By only about 10 per cent.

65 Acetazolamide:
  (a) Causes pupillary dilatation, to accelerate drainage of the aqueous humour.
  (b) Has anticonvulsant properties.
  (c) Causes an alkaline diuresis.
  (d) Is contraindicated in the presence of cysteine renal stones.
  (e) Is extensively metabolized into sulphanilamide.

66 Thiazides:
  (a) Are weak carbonic anhydrase inhibitors.
  (b) Cause an alkaline diuresis.
  (c) Accelerate calcium loss from the body.
  (d) Induce hyperuricaemia.
  (e) Accelerate magnesium loss from the body.

67 Bumetanide:
  (a) Causes less potassium loss than thiazide diuretics.
  (b) Has a shorter duration of action than chlorthalidone.
  (c) Is less potent on a weight for weight basis than frusemide.
  (d) Administration may cause musculoskeletal pain and muscle spasm.
  (e) Has aldosterone antagonist properties.

68 Ethacrynic acid:
  (a) Acts primarily at the proximal tubule of the loop of Henle.
  (b) Accelerates calcium loss from the body.
  (c) Is less likely to cause gastrointestinal bleeding than frusemide.
  (d) Does not exacerbate diabetes.
  (e) Is ototoxic.

69 Mannitol:
  (a) Is metabolized to sorbitol which itself has a diuretic action.
  (b) Undergoes active tubular secretion with minimal reabsorption.
  (c) Is hypotonic as a 25 per cent solution and may induce haemolysis if administered at a rate greater than 3 g/minute.
  (d) Has been used in the treatment of the unconscious eclamptic patient.
  (e) May reduce the severity of ischaemic renal impairment if administered before the insult.

70 Frusemide:
  (a) Like bumetanide may produce hyperuricaemia.
  (b) Is more ototoxic than bumetanide.
  (c) Is less likely to induce hyperglycaemia than bumetanide.
  (d) Has no effect on plasma renin.
  (e) Is synergistic with bumetanide in cases of resistant oedema.

71 Amiloride:
  (a) Acts as a diuretic by inhibition of sodium transport in the distal parts of the nephron.
  (b) Administration may give rise to hyperglycaemia in much the same way as thiazides.
  (c) May give rise to some degree of azotaemia.
  (d) Accelerates the loss of magnesium from the body.
  (e) Can give rise to hyperkalaemia.

65 (a) **False**   It decreases the production of the aqueous humour.
   (b) **True**   By a direct action on the central nervous system.
   (c) **True**   Leading to a metabolic acidosis which tends to limit its effects.
   (d) **False**   Although prolonged use can result in calculi an alkaline urine is useful in the treatment of cysteine stones.
   (e) **False**   Acetazolamide is not metabolized.

66 (a) **True**
   (b) **False**   Chloride or bicarbonate loss accompany the sodium loss.
   (c) **False**   They may be useful in the treatment for hypercalciuria.
   (d) **True**   By enhanced reabsorption of urate in the proximal tubule and inhibition of tubular excretion.
   (e) **True**   With possible occurrence of hypomagnesaemia.

67 (a) **False**   The potassium excretion is similar.
   (b) **True**
   (c) **False**   It is more potent.
   (d) **True**
   (e) **False**   It is a high-ceiling or loop diuretic.

68 (a) **False**   It acts primarily at the ascending limb of the loop.
   (b) **True**   In proportion to the sodium excretion.
   (c) **False**   It is more likely.
   (d) **False**
   (e) **True**   Deafness, tinnitus and vertigo may occur.

69 (a) **False**   It is excreted unchanged.
   (b) **False**   It undergoes glomerular filtration.
   (c) **False**   It is hypertonic, the limit on the rate of administration is true however.
   (d) **True**   On the basis that many of these patients have cerebral oedema.
   (e) **True**   The osmotic effect of mannitol inhibits water reabsorption maintaining an adequate flow of relatively dilute urine, which is an important factor in the prevention of renal damage.

70 (a) **True**
   (b) **True**   But ethacrynic acid is the most ototoxic of the 'loop diuretics'. The damage is worse if an aminoglycoside antibiotic is being administered simultaneously.
   (c) **False**   Glucose tolerance is better with bumetanide.
   (d) **False**   The renal secretion of renin is increased resulting in a redistribution of the renal blood flow. The effect can be inhibited by prostaglandin inhibitors such as indomethacin.
   (e) **False**   There is no synergism in the effects of the two. Moreover, administering the two together has no therapeutic advantage.

71 (a) **True**
   (b) **False**   Amiloride does not cause hyperglycaemia.
   (c) **True**   This is not thought to be directly related to electrolyte and water imbalance. It is also reversible.
   (d) **False**   It is of value because it does not accelerate magnesium loss and so may reduce cardiac irregularities due to hypomagnesaemia.
   (e) **True**   Toxicity due to hyperkalaemia is a real possibility with amiloride and other potassium-sparing diuretics.

72 Poor response to diuretic therapy:
  (a) Occurs if the glomerular filtration rate (GFR) is below 15 ml/minute.
  (b) May occur in hypokalaemia.
  (c) Occurs in hyponatraemia.
  (d) May occur during lithium therapy.
  (e) May occur during therapy for rheumatoid arthritis.

73 Urinary retention may result from:
  (a) Ephedrine.
  (b) Imipramine.
  (c) Distigmine.
  (d) Indoramin.
  (e) Atropine.

Drugs and the respiratory system

74 Ketotifen:
  (a) Protects against exercise-induced bronchoconstriction.
  (b) Attenuates the effects of seasonal asthma.
  (c) Is useful in the treatment of atopic dermatitis.
  (d) Has bronchodilating properties roughly equivalent to ipratropium bromide.
  (e) Can lead to agitation especially in small children.

75 Salmeterol:
  (a) Is a salbutamol prodrug.
  (b) Is more potent than salbutamol.
  (c) Is more lipid soluble than salbutamol
  (d) Has the advantage of being free from producing muscle tremor.
  (e) Has inhibitory effects against inflammatory responses.

76 Exogenous lung surfactant (colfosceril palmitate):
  (a) Rapidly improves pulmonary gas exchange in premature infants.
  (b) Rapidly improves lung compliance in premature infants.
  (c) Impedes oedema formation in the lung.
  (d) Stabilizes small airways.
  (e) May play a role in the transport of mucous.

72 (a) **True**   Few diuretics work well at such low filtration rates.
   (b) **True**   Particularly in severe hypokalaemia.
   (c) **True**
   (d) **True**
   (e) **True**   Due to the effect of non-steroidal anti-inflammatory drug therapy.

73 (a) **True**   Particularly in men with prostatic hypertrophy.
   (b) **True**   Due to its anticholinergic effects. Imipramine is used in the treat-
                     ment of enuresis.
   (c) **False**   It is an anticholinesterase agent used in the prevention of urinary
                     retention.
   (d) **False**   It increases the urinary flow rate by action at the postsynaptic
                     alpha$_1$-adrenoceptors. It is sometimes used in the management of
                     outflow obstruction due to benign prostatic hypertrophy.
   (e) **True**

---

74 (a) **False**
   (b) **True**   But it must be given several weeks in advance.
   (c) **True**   Ketotifen has a potent and long lasting antihistamine action.
   (d) **False**   It is not a bronchodilator but it can attenuate the tachyphylaxis to
                     beta$_2$-adrenoceptor agonist bronchodilators.
   (e) **False**   It is very well tolerated especially in small children. The main side-
                     effect is sedation.

75 (a) **False**   This drug was produced in an attempt to make a long acting
                     bronchodilator. It has been created by manipulation of the
                     salbutamol molecule in which the polar phenylethanolamine
                     group interacts with the beta-adrenoceptor while the long non-polar
                     side-chain interacts with the cell membrane to give a long half-life to
                     the drug–receptor complex.
   (b) **True**   In addition it is a highly selective drug.
   (c) **True**
   (d) **False**
   (e) **True**   Salmeterol has been shown to inhibit the release of thromboxane
                     A$_2$ from human alveolar macrophages. Caution should be exer-
                     cised, however, since the use of such drugs may mask the wors-
                     ening of the disease process.

76 (a) **True**   This drug is now available for wider use following promising trials.
   (b) **False**   Improvement in oxygenation is probably due to other properties of
                     the drug such as reduction of interstitial lung water and prevention
                     of alveolar flooding. In the normal course of events surface tension
                     forces at the alveolar air–fluid interface would promote alveolar
                     flooding were it not for endogenous surfactant.
   (c) **True**   (See (b) above).
   (d) **True**   This is true for both the exogenous as well as the endogenous
                     surfactant even though the latter, which is made in the alveoli
                     has to be delivered to the bronchial system where it stabilizes the
                     airways and promotes the transport of mucous.
   (e) **True**   (See (d) above).

77 Racemic adrenaline:
  (a) Consists of L-adrenaline.
  (b) Is useful in controlling bronchial congestion because of its beta-adrenoceptor stimulating effects.
  (c) Is a potent mast cell stabilizer.
  (d) Has the advantage of being effective by the oral route.
  (e) Can lead to tolerance to its own effects.

78 Salbutamol:
  (a) Is as likely as isoprenaline to produce tachycardia.
  (b) Is associated with hyperkalaemia.
  (c) Unlike ritodrine has no effect on the uterus.
  (d) Induced bronchodilatation may show tachyphylaxis.
  (e) Induced tremor can show tachyphylaxis.

79 Terfenadine:
  (a) Is as sedative as chlorpheniramine.
  (b) Has no affinity for H_2-receptors
  (c) Has significant anticholinergic activity
  (d) Potentiates the effects of alcohol.
  (e) May have a role in the treatment of chronic urticaria.

80 Methylxanthines:
  (a) Exert all their effects due to phosphodiesterase inhibition.
  (b) Stimulate the medullary respiratory centre.
  (c) Increase the secretion of gastric acid.
  (d) Have significant antihistaminic effects.
  (e) Have no effect on the sensitivity of the medullary centres to the stimulant effects of carbon dioxide.

81 Theophylline toxicity:
  (a) Is manifest at plasma levels 20–40 mg/litre.
  (b) Usually results in nausea.
  (c) May result in hypotonia.
  (d) Can be avoided in congestive heart failure by decreasing the loading dose.
  (e) May be treated by charcoal haemoperfusion.

77 (a) **False** It is a mixture of equal parts of D- and L-isomers of adrenaline. Naturally occurring adrenaline is found only in the L-form.

(b) **False** It does reduce congestion, however, this is because of its alpha-adrenergic effects producing vasoconstriction of the bronchial mucosal vasculature.

(c) **True**

(d) **False** It is almost totally ineffective by this route.

(e) **True** Due to so called 'down regulation' of adrenoceptors.

78 (a) **False** It is a selective agent.

(b) **False** It may produce hypokalaemia.

(c) **False** Both agents relax the uterus.

(d) **True**

(e) **True**

79 (a) **False** This is a selective H_1-receptor antagonist which has little influence on central H_1-receptors unlike chlorpheniramine.

(b) **True** It is a specific H_1-receptor antagonist with no H_2-receptor or beta- or alpha-adrenoceptor blocking effects. It may have some antiserotonin activity as well.

(c) **False**

(d) **False** Studies have failed to show this with alcohol or diazepam.

(e) **True** Because of its lack of sedative effects it is also acceptable to patients. Astemizole is slower and even longer acting.

80 (a) **False** While the ability of these compounds to inhibit phosphodiesterase is often quoted, significant inhibition is in fact usually seen at plasma levels, that are usually toxic. Actions on sympathetic activity, antagonism of adenosine and inflammatory mediator release may contribute to its effects.

(b) **True** They have been assessed for use in neonatal sleep apnoea problems.

(c) **True** They increase the secretion of both gastric acid and pepsin. A warning to excessive tea drinkers perhaps!

(d) **False**

(e) **False** The sensitivity of the medullary centres is increased.

81 (a) **True** Theophylline has a narrow therapeutic range between 10–20 mg/litre.

(b) **True** Especially on chronic administration when gut symptoms such as nausea, vomiting and abdominal pain may predominate. Theophylline can both stimulate the medullary vomiting centre and cause gastric irritation.

(c) **False** Hyper-reflexia is usually present.

(d) **False** Not the loading dose but the maintenance dose, as the clearance of theophylline decreases in congestive heart failure.

(e) **True**

82 Sodium cromoglycate:
   (a) Antagonises the effects of the chemical mediators in asthma.
   (b) Has useful bronchodilating properties.
   (c) Is of little benefit in late onset asthma.
   (d) Is not effective in the prevention of exercise-induced asthma.
   (e) Has no histamine-receptor blocking properties.

83 Ipratropium bromide:
   (a) Is a more lipid soluble derivative of atropine.
   (b) Unlike atropine does not inhibit mucociliary clearance.
   (c) Acts more rapidly than beta-adrenoceptor agonists in the relief of asthmatic symptoms.
   (d) Is contraindicated in patients with glaucoma.
   (e) Acts synergistically with salbutamol.

84 Nedocromil sodium:
   (a) Shows greater anti-inflammatory effects than cromoglycate.
   (b) Is ineffective against exercise-induced asthma.
   (c) Is as potent as inhaled steroids in the treatment of asthma.
   (d) Suffers from the disadvantage of not being well absorbed after oral administration.
   (e) Causes sedation.

Drugs used in anaesthesia

85 Thiopentone:
   (a) Offers significant cerebral protection if used in resuscitation from cardiac arrest.
   (b) Is useful for cerebral protection for valvular surgery using extracorporeal circulation.
   (c) In clinically used anaesthetic doses produces the same degree of reduction in cerebral metabolic oxygen requirement as cooling to 28°C.
   (d) Is a free radical scavenger.
   (e) Administration over a prolonged period of time is beneficial in controlling intracranial pressure after head injury.

86 The following may be associated with convulsant activity in susceptible individuals:
   (a) Etomidate.
   (b) Fentanyl.
   (c) Diazepam.
   (d) Ketamine.
   (e) Propofol.

87 Among the barbiturate anaesthetic agents:
   (a) Thiopentone has been linked to convulsions in non-epileptic patients.
   (b) Thiopentone infusions have been used for days to control status epilepticus.
   (c) Methohexitone has not been shown to provoke convulsions in patients with generalized convulsive disorders.
   (d) Methohexitone in low doses is useful in producing electroencephalographic evidence of seizures in temporal lobe epilepsy.
   (e) Thiopentone will induce seizure activity in temporal lobe epilepsy.

82 (a) **False**   It prevents the release of histamine and other mediators of the inflammatory response rather than antagonize their effect.
 (b) **False**   It is not a smooth muscle relaxant, although it was discovered during the search for such a drug.
 (c) **True**
 (d) **False**   It is effective but only when used well in advance.
 (e) **True**

83 (a) **False**   It is less lipid soluble with little systemic absorption and central side-effects. It has been designed to antagonize the cholinergically-mediated bronchoconstriction, and, as such, may be of benefit when there is tolerance to beta$_2$-receptor agonists.
 (b) **True**   For unexplained reasons.
 (c) **False**   It is the other way round.
 (d) **False**   The drug is poorly absorbed.
 (e) **True**   It results in prolongation of the action of salbutamol.

84 (a) **True**
 (b) **False**
 (c) **False**   It may at best be dose-sparing.
 (d) **True**   It is useful mostly by inhalation.
 (e) **False**

---

85 (a) **False**   It really needs to be given prophylactically.
 (b) **True**   This is the only situation where there is proven benefit.
 (c) **False**
 (d) **True**
 (e) **False**   Also, not only is it therapeutically of no benefit, but also results in marked cardiovascular depression.

86 (a) **True**   However myoclonus following etomidate is subcortical in origin.
 (b) **False**   Although extremely large doses (not used in humans) may produce convulsions in dogs.
 (c) **True**   This paradoxical action is usually restricted to patients with Lennox Gastaut syndrome (a form of secondary generalized epilepsy), it does not occur in normal individuals.
 (d) **True**
 (e) **False**

87 (a) **False**
 (b) **True**   At the risk of cardiovascular depression.
 (c) **True**   Although it will do so in patients with epilepsy.
 (d) **True**   Low-dose methohexitone has been used to activate and define epileptogenic foci during temporal lobectomy.
 (e) **False**

88 Thiopentone:
   (a) Has a terminal elimination half-life, which is approximately three times its distribution half-life.
   (b) Will show zero order kinetics at high doses.
   (c) Crosses the blood–brain barrier in much reduced quantities in acidosis.
   (d) Shows a prolonged elimination half-life in renal failure.
   (e) Has a terminal elimination half-life in children about half that in adults.

89 Ketamine:
   (a) Is solubilized in ethylene glycol.
   (b) Decreases the pulmonary artery pressure in spite of increasing the systemic arterial pressure.
   (c) Exists as enantiomers which differ in anaesthetic potency.
   (d) Is not effective when given orally because of extensive first-pass metabolism.
   (e) Has active metabolites with ketamine-like effects.

90 Ketamine:
   (a) Has no analgesic effects at subanaesthetic doses.
   (b) Has no effect on intrathecal administration.
   (c) Causes both sensory and motor block when used for intravenous regional analgesia.
   (d) Increases systemic vascular resistance.
   (e) Causes sialorrhoea.

91 Propofol:
   (a) When injected into a large antecubital vein, shows a similar incidence of pain on injection as thiopentone.
   (b) Results in apnoea with much the same frequency as thiopentone.
   (c) Has a similar initial distribution half-life as thiopentone.
   (d) Has a rate of clearance twice that of thiopentone.
   (e) Is less protein bound than thiopentone.

92 Propofol:
   (a) Is contraindicated in porphyria.
   (b) Is approximately half as potent as thiopentone.
   (c) Produces retrograde amnesia.
   (d) Causes more cardiovascular depression than thiopentone.
   (e) Has no antianalgesic effect.

93 Propofol:
   (a) Is 98 per cent protein bound in the blood stream.
   (b) Clearance is markedly reduced in cirrhosis of liver.
   (c) Pharmacokinetics are not significantly altered in renal failure.
   (d) Levels may be higher in the presence of fentanyl.
   (e) Has a markedly prolonged elimination half-life in the elderly.

88 (a) **False** It is very much longer than that (10–12 hours).
   (b) **True** Hence the very high plasma levels which cause myocardial depression after prolonged infusions.
   (c) **False** The passage is increased.
   (d) **False** Although reduced plasma protein binding leads to higher levels of the free drug and a larger volume of distribution, increased clearance results in little overall change.
   (e) **True** Because of a higher rate of clearance.

89 (a) **False** It is a water-soluble agent.
   (b) **False** Both are increased.
   (c) **True** Commercial ketamine is a mixture of these.
   (d) **False** Although it does show a first-pass effect.
   (e) **True** Norketamine has one third the potency of ketamine.

90 (a) **False**
   (b) **False** Both sensory and motor block are produced, albeit of short duration.
   (c) **True** The patients may, however, get anaesthetized when the tourniquet is released.
   (d) **True**
   (e) **True**

91 (a) **True** Both produce less pain than methohexitone.
   (b) **True** Although propofol-induced apnoea is longer.
   (c) **True** 2–8 minutes.
   (d) **False** It is at least seven times.
   (e) **False** It is more protein bound.

92 (a) **False** Propofol has been used in porphyria without adverse effects.
   (b) **False** Thiopentone is half as potent.
   (c) **False** It has no such effects.
   (d) **True**
   (e) **True** Unlike the barbiturates.

93 (a) **True**
   (b) **False** Although propofol is metabolized by glucuronidation or sulphation before renal excretion.
   (c) **True**
   (d) **True** An effect also seen with etomidate.
   (e) **False** Although the rate of clearance is somewhat lower.

94 Etomidate:
  (a) Is a carboxylated ether derivative.
  (b) Is not water soluble.
  (c) Administration is complicated by significant thrombophlebitis.
  (d) Is not highly protein bound.
  (e) Is 98 per cent excreted as inactive metabolites in the urine.

95 Etomidate:
  (a) Administration results in an increase of intracranial pressure secondary to myoclonus.
  (b) Administration produces an increase in intraocular pressure secondary to myoclonus.
  (c) Liberates histamine only in minimal amounts in the young.
  (d) Causes minimal changes in systemic vascular resistance.
  (e) Causes a decrease in heart rate.

96 Etomidate:
  (a) Has a similar incidence of coughing and hiccough to methohexitone.
  (b) Myoclonus is not decreased by pretreatment with benzodiazepines
  (c) Causes less respiratory depression than methohexitone.
  (d) Causes an irreversible inhibition of 11 beta-hydroxylation reactions leading to an inhibition of steroidogenesis.
  (e) Kinetics are unaltered during high-dose fentanyl anaesthesia.

97 The following are true about the structure–activity relationship of barbiturates:

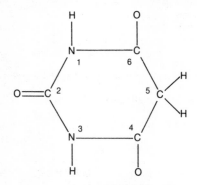

Barbituric acid

  (a) Adding a phenyl group to barbituric acid at C5 confers anticonvulsant activity.
  (b) An alkyl side chain at C5 is unrelated to hypnotic activity.
  (c) Replacing oxygen with sulphur at C2 results in enhanced lipid solubility and a rapid onset of effect.
  (d) Methylation of the nitrogen at C1 results in a rapid hypnotic action but also excitatory phenomena.
  (e) Methylation at position C1 and replacing oxygen with sulphur at position C2 results in thiopentone.

94 (a) **False** It is a carboxylated imidazole derivative.
   (b) **False** It is water soluble, but is formulated in propylene glycol because it is unstable in aqueous solution.
   (c) **True** This may be related to the high osmolarity of the preparation; 4640 mOsmol/litre.
   (d) **False** It is more than 75 per cent protein bound.
   (e) **True** Following hepatic metabolism.

95 (a) **False** Bolus administration results in a decrease in intracranial pressure.
   (b) **False** Etomidate reduces the intraocular pressure.
   (c) **True** Relative to the other induction agents.
   (d) **True**
   (e) **False** The heart rate usually increases.

96 (a) **True**
   (b) **False**
   (c) **True**
   (d) **False** Not irreversible! Etomidate inhibits cytochrome P450 to prevent the resynthesis of ascorbic acid, loss of which leads to a failure of steroidogenesis. (Humans of course need ascorbic acid as a vitamin, many animals synthesize it themselves.)
   (e) **False** The rate of clearance of etomidate is reduced.

97 (a) **True** As with phenobarbitone.
   (b) **False** If the side chain, however, is too long, excitatory phenomena appear.
   (c) **True**
   (d) **True** Methohexitone is an example.
   (e) **False** These are not the characteristics of thiopentone. Methylated thiobarbiturates although potent and rapid acting have an unacceptable incidence of excitatory activity for clinical use.

98 The following drugs can prolong non-depolarizing neuromuscular blockade:
   (a) Neomycin.
   (b) Lignocaine.
   (c) Theophylline.
   (d) Azathioprine.
   (e) Magnesium.

99 The effect of tubocurarine is potentiated by:
   (a) Acidosis.
   (b) Alkalosis.
   (c) Mild hypothermia
   (d) Severe hypothermia (less than 30°C)
   (e) Hypokalaemia.

100 Suxamethonium:
   (a) Will trigger malignant hyperthermia only in humans.
   (b) Has no effect on autonomic ganglia.
   (c) Induced myalgia has no relation to the degree of fasciculations.
   (d) Has no active metabolites.
   (e) Induced release of muscle enzymes is more common in the presence of halothane anaesthesia.

101 Atracurium:
   (a) Is a bisquaternary aminosteroid with an intermediate duration of action.
   (b) Has the advantage of being completely metabolized by the process of Hofmann elimination.
   (c) Produces cutaneous flushing in a dose-related manner.
   (d) Unlike vecuronium may increase the intraocular pressure.
   (e) Requirements are greater in patients with significant burns.

102 Nitrous oxide:
   (a) Supports combustion.
   (b) Allows more rapid conduction of sound than oxygen.
   (c) Has a blood–gas partition coefficient of 1.
   (d) Is more fat soluble than halothane.
   (e) Has a critical temperature of 36.43°C.

103 Nitrous oxide:
   (a) Has minimal effect on ventilation when administered in a 50 per cent concentration in oxygen.
   (b) Is a direct myocardial depressant.
   (c) Is a stimulant of the sympathetic nervous system.
   (d) Is metabolized to nitric oxide in the body.
   (e) Is active at opiate receptors.

98 (a) **True**   Possibly by a presynaptic effect.
(b) **True**
(c) **False** It produces an antagonism.
(d) **False** It antagonizes the block.
(e) **True**

99 (a) **True**   Whether metabolic or respiratory.
(b) **False**
(c) **False**
(d) **True**
(e) **True**

100 (a) **False** There is nothing special about humans in this respect.
(b) **False**
(c) **True**   The correlation between the two is poor.
(d) **False** Succinylmonocholine may actually exert some of its effect.
(e) **True**   Both in animal models and in man.

101 (a) **False** It is a benzylisoquinoline derivative which resembles the steroidal agent vecuronium in its intermediate duration of action.
(b) **False** This process accounts for about 40–50 per cent of metabolism of atracurium, non-specific esterases and organ uptake account for the rest.
(c) **True**   Higher doses may also produce systemic effects of histamine liberation.
(d) **False** Neither agent raises the intraocular pressure.
(e) **True**

102 (a) **True**   In addition it decomposes into nitrogen and oxygen at temperatures above 450°C.
(b) **False** It is the reverse. This principle allows the use of a whistle to distinguish between the two gases.
(c) **False** It is 0.47 indicating low solubility in blood. A low solubility facilitates a rapid induction of anaesthesia.
(d) **False**
(e) **True**

103 (a) **True**
(b) **True**   In *in vitro* preparations. In man the effects are more complex because nitrous oxide is rarely used as a sole anaesthetic. Some reduction in cardiac output is observed when nitrous oxide is added to anaesthesia with morphine, even though the arterial pressure is maintained.
(c) **True**
(d) **False** Nitrous oxide is not metabolized.
(e) **True**   But not all its analgesic activity is explained this way.

104 Enflurane:
   (a) Is a halogenated hydrocarbon in contrast to isoflurane, which is a halogen-
       ated ether.
   (b) Has a higher MAC than cyclopropane.
   (c) Is stable in ultraviolet light.
   (d) Has a boiling point of 56.5°C.
   (e) Has a higher oil–gas partition coefficient than halothane.

105 Isoflurane:
   (a) Has virtually the same vapour pressure as halothane.
   (b) Has the highest blood–gas partition coefficient amongst the commonly
       used anaesthetic agents with the exception of ether and methoxyflurane.
   (c) Is non-flammable in air but flammable in oxygen.
   (d) Does not require a preservative.
   (e) Potentiates muscle relaxants to a lesser extent than halothane.

106 Halothane:
   (a) Produces less myocardial depression than isoflurane.
   (b) Increases the refractory period of the atrioventricular junction more than
       enflurane.
   (c) Administration produces a dose-related decrease in left ventricular filling
       pressure.
   (d) Anaesthesia is associated with a rise in right atrial pressure.
   (e) Produces less cardiovascular depression during spontaneous ventilation.

107 Central nervous system excitability:
   (a) Is rare after isoflurane.
   (b) May sometimes be observed in the postoperative period after halothane
       anaesthesia.
   (c) With enflurane is dose-independent.
   (d) Is common after enflurane in the presence of normocapnia.
   (e) Is not related to the cerebral vasodilating effects of volatile agents.

108 Hepatotoxicity:
   (a) Following halothane has been demonstrated more often in the presence of
       drug-induced enzyme induction in animal models.
   (b) With halothane is more common in females.
   (c) With enflurane is 50 per cent as common as with halothane.
   (d) Is not a feature of isoflurane.
   (e) With halothane is unrelated to ethnic origin.

109 Halothane:
   (a) Is not associated with hepatitis in children.
   (b) Never causes hepatitis on first exposure.
   (c) Related hepatitis does not occur if repeat administration is avoided
       within 3 months of an uneventful first exposure.
   (d) Hepatitis is commoner in those with pre-existing compensated liver disease.
   (e) Is commoner in patients with preoperative enzyme induction.

104 (a) **False**   Both are ethers.
  (b) **False**   The MAC of enflurane is 1.68 and that of cyclopropane 9.2.
  (c) **True**
  (d) **True**
  (e) **False**   Oil–gas partition coefficients of enflurane and halothane are 98.5 and 224 respectively.

105 (a) **True**   Approximately 240 mmHg at 20°C for both.
  (b) **False**   It is only 1.4 as against 1.9 for enflurane and 2.3 for halothane. The slow induction sometimes observed with it is due to its pungent smell.
  (c) **False**
  (d) **True**   It is quite stable.
  (e) **False**

106 (a) **False**   It is the other way.
  (b) **True**
  (c) **False**   Progressive depression of left ventricular function results in an increase in left ventricular filling pressure.
  (d) **True**
  (e) **True**   Because of increased sympathetic activity because of elevated carbon dioxide levels and maintenance of a negative intrathoracic pressure.

107 (a) **True**
  (b) **False**   'Halothane shakes' are not central nervous system excitability.
  (c) **False**   It is dose-related and is observed with increasing depth of anaesthesia.
  (d) **False**   It is more common during hypocapnia and when using high-inspired enflurane concentrations.
  (e) **True**

108 (a) **True**   Such as in phenobarbitone-treated rats.
  (b) **True**   By a ratio of 2:1.
  (c) **False**   Although there are some reports, the incidence is very low.
  (d) **True**   For the time being.
  (e) **False**   Genetics do seem to play some part, with a case cluster in a few Mexican-Americans. HLA antigen DR2 may be more common in patients showing jaundice.

109 (a) **False**   It is just less common at the extremes of age.
  (b) **False**   Cases after the first exposure have been reported.
  (c) **False**   There is no safe period as such, although it is generally agreed that an interval of more than 3 months is safe.
  (d) **False**   There is no correlation between pre-existing liver disease and halothane hepatitis. Obviously, however, it is good practice to avoid the use of halothane in these groups for other reasons.
  (e) **False**   Although there is good evidence of this in animal models.

110 Enflurane:
   (a) Causes dose-related changes in liver transaminases.
   (b) Is relatively contraindicated in chronic renal failure.
   (c) Is relatively contraindicated in patients treated with isoniazid.
   (d) Produces much less free fluoride than halothane when used for long procedures in the obese.
   (e) Is not associated with malignant hyperpyrexia.

111 Desflurane:
   (a) Is a fluorinated methyl ether similar to isoflurane.
   (b) Is unstable in the presence of soda lime.
   (c) Has a MAC of about 1.5.
   (d) Is minimally biotransformed.
   (e) Shows faster recovery from anaesthesia than all other volatile agents.

112 Sevoflurane:
   (a) Is a fluorinated hydrocarbon similar to halothane.
   (b) Has a MAC of about 2.
   (c) Causes depression of cardiac output similar to halothane.
   (d) Causes respiratory stimulation.
   (e) May be associated with muscle rigidity on induction.

113 Isoflurane:
   (a) Increases the cerebral blood flow to the same extent as enflurane when administered at concentrations of greater than 1.5 MAC.
   (b) Depresses cerebral oxygen consumption to the same extent as sodium nitroprusside.
   (c) Preserves the responsiveness of the cerebral vasculature to carbon dioxide more than enflurane.
   (d) Has little effect on pulmonary vascular resistance.
   (e) Among the commonly used inhalational agents has the least effect on uterine muscle.

General and local analgesic drugs

114 Morphine:
   (a) Inhibits the release of adrenocorticotropic hormone (ACTH).
   (b) Stimulates the release of antidiuretic hormone (ADH).
   (c) Stimulates the Edinger-Westphal nucleus.
   (d) Shifts the 'ventilation response curve' to carbon dioxide to the left.
   (e) Antagonizes the effects of both endogenous and exogenous substance P.

115 Morphine:
   (a) Increases gastric emptying time.
   (b) Increases hydrochloric acid secretion in the stomach.
   (c) Decreases peristalsis.
   (d) Decreases ileocolic and anal sphincter tone.
   (e) Increases the likelihood of oesophageal reflux.

110 (a) **False** These are not dose-related.
  (b) **True** Because it is biotransformed to yield free inorganic fluoride with plasma levels in some obese patients of 50 μmol/litre. Free fluoride is nephrotoxic.
  (c) **True** This specifically induces the biotransformation of enflurane to free fluoride.
  (d) **False** Even though halothane undergoes more metabolism than enflurane it yields less fluoride.
  (e) **False**

111 (a) **True** It also shares properties such as being non-flammable and non-explosive.
  (b) **False** It is stable and will need to be used employing a closed circuit because of the high cost.
  (c) **False** Its MAC is approximately 6.
  (d) **True**
  (e) **True** The drug is relatively insoluble with a blood–gas partition co-efficient of about 0.42. The induction is also quick and smooth as it has a pleasant odour and is non-irritable.

112 (a) **False** It is a halogenated methyl isopropyl ether.
  (b) **True**
  (c) **False** It is less marked than with halothane but more marked than with isoflurane.
  (d) **False** There is dose-related respiratory depression.
  (e) **True** Particularly in children.

113 (a) **True** However at lower concentrations isoflurane has less effect.
  (b) **False** isoflurane produces greater reduction.
  (c) **True**
  (d) **False** In general all inhalational agents depress hypoxic pulmonary vasoconstriction.
  (e) **True** At equipotent doses.

---

114 (a) **True** Morphine can both stimulate and inhibit various parts of the brain.
  (b) **True**
  (c) **True** A direct action causes this stimulation and instigates miosis.
  (d) **False** The displacement is to the right with a reduction in the slope of the curve.
  (e) **True** Morphine not only antagonizes the effects of endogenous substance P but may also inhibit its release. The antagonism of exogenous substance P is by a slightly different mechanism.

115 (a) **True** As gastric motility is decreased
  (b) **False**
  (c) **True** Although the tone of the small intestine increases.
  (d) **False** The tone is actually increased, delaying the passage of gut contents, and so increasing water reabsorption.
  (e) **True** There is decreased gastric motility; this can be a risk factor in anaesthesia.

116 Following morphine administration:
   (a) Only 30 per cent of an orally given dose reaches the systemic circulation in a healthy adult.
   (b) The bioavailability by the buccal route is greater than by the oral route.
   (c) The absorption is almost 90 per cent complete within 10 minutes after intramuscular administration.
   (d) The elimination half-life is considerably prolonged even in mild cirrhosis of the liver.
   (e) The metabolism is unaltered in renal failure.

117 Diamorphine:
   (a) Is a faster acting analgesic than morphine.
   (b) Unlike morphine is not subject to extensive hepatic first-pass metabolism.
   (c) Has no active metabolites.
   (d) In a dose of 20 mg is equivalent to 20 mg of papaveretum.
   (e) Given via the intrathecal route is just as likely as morphine to cause delayed respiratory depression.

118 Pentazocine:
   (a) Is about a third as potent as morphine.
   (b) Is as useful as morphine in the treatment of the pain of myocardial infarction.
   (c) In equianalgesic doses to morphine is more likely to cause euphoria.
   (d) Can be used to antagonize the respiratory depressant effects of fentanyl.
   (e) Causes the same degree of respiratory depression as morphine in equianalgesic doses.

119 Pethidine:
   (a) Has one-tenth the potency of morphine.
   (b) Is a vagotonic opioid.
   (c) Is the least likely of the opioids to cross the placenta.
   (d) In equianalgesic doses to morphine has less effect on gastric emptying.
   (e) Is more likely than morphine to lead to convulsions in overdose.

116 (a) **True**   High hepatic extraction occurs resulting in significant first-pass metabolism.

   (b) **False**   Mean bioavailability is only about 19 per cent after buccal morphine, the technique also has poor patient acceptance.

   (c) **False**   This requires about 45 minutes.

   (d) **False**   Morphine is metabolized by hepatic glucuronidation to morphine-3-glucuronide and morphine-6-glucuronide. This reaction is relatively well preserved until severe hepatic impairment has taken place. However, the bioavailability after oral administration may increase.

   (e) **False**   The metabolites mentioned above are excreted in the urine, and morphine-6-glucuronide in particular has pharmacological effects similar to those of morphine. Plasma protein binding of morphine is also reduced in renal disease resulting in immediate greater effect after injection.

117 (a) **True**   Replacing the two hydroxyl groups in morphine with acetyl groups results in enhanced lipid solubility and more rapid onset of analgesia, but not necessarily a greater effect.

   (b) **False**   The drug is extensively metabolized to monoacetyl morphine and morphine; as a result morphine is found in plasma after oral administration of diamorphine.

   (c) **False**   Monoacetyl morphine and morphine are pharmacologically active.

   (d) **False**   Papaveretum is a mixture of opium alkaloids standardized to contain 50 per cent anhydrous morphine.

   (e) **False**   Delayed respiratory depression is a feature of less lipid soluble compounds.

118 (a) **True**   It has about a half to a third the activity of morphine.

   (b) **False**   Pentazocine, unlike morphine, can cause increase in heart rate, blood pressure and plasma catecholamines causing an increase in the cardiac workload.

   (c) **False**   It is associated with dysphoria, being an agonist at kappa and sigma opioid receptors and a weak antagonist at mu receptors.

   (d) **True**   It uses the weak mu receptor antagonist properties.

   (e) **True**   There may be a plateau effect, however, to the degree of respiratory depression.

119 (a) **True**   As it is more lipid soluble than morphine, however, it will have a faster onset of effect.

   (b) **False**   If anything it is vagolytic, having been derived from a number of atropine-like compounds.

   (c) **False**   Its placental transfer is virtually unrestricted even to the extent that the fetal blood pethidine concentration may exceed that in the maternal blood. Pentazocine is the exception among the opioids in that its placental transfer is less extensive.

   (d) **False**   Gastric emptying is slowed considerably leading to delayed absorption of other substances from the gastrointestinal tract.

   (e) **True**   This is thought to be because of its metabolite norpethidine. It is also more likely to cause problems in the presence of monoamine oxidase inhibitors.

120 Extradurally or intrathecally administered opioids:
  (a) Are effective because they resemble local anaesthetics in their physico-chemical properties.
  (b) Have a duration of action directly proportional to their lipid solubility.
  (c) Abolish vasoconstrictor responses.
  (d) May cause hallucinations.
  (e) May suppress polysynaptic flexion reflexes.

121 Concerning intrathecal and extradural administration of opioids:
  (a) The incidence of urinary retention is similar with both routes of administration.
  (b) Pruritus is more common after intrathecal administration.
  (c) Emetic effects are related to the total dose of opioid and not to the route of administration.
  (d) Early and brief respiratory depression is a feature of lipophilic opioids.
  (e) Extradural opioids produce better analgesia in the first stage of labour.

122 Fentanyl:
  (a) Has a longer distribution half-life than morphine.
  (b) Has a shorter elimination half-life than alfentanil.
  (c) Is much more lipid soluble than alfentanil.
  (d) Has a similar pKa value to alfentanil.
  (e) Has a similar volume of distribution to alfentanil.

123 Alfentanil:
  (a) Produces more respiratory depression than an equianalgesic dose of fentanyl.
  (b) Induces more bradycardia than an equianalgesic dose of fentanyl.
  (c) Produces a more rapid onset of rigidity than equianalgesic doses of fentanyl.
  (d) May produce more nausea than fentanyl.
  (e) Is too short acting to induce dependence.

124 Sufentanil:
  (a) Has half the potency of fentanyl.
  (b) Shows far fewer side-effects than other potent opioids in equianalgesic doses.
  (c) Is slower in onset of action than alfentanil.
  (d) Is more rapid in onset of action than fentanyl.
  (e) Has shorter distribution and elimination half-lives than fentanyl.

120 (a) **True**   Local anaesthetics and opioids are very similar in their physico-chemical properties.

(b) **False**   It is the opposite. It is a feature of the speed of action.

(c) **False**   These act at specific opioid receptors rather than at the sympathetic nerves.

(d) **True**   Hallucinations have been reported after high doses have been administered intrathecally.

(e) **True**   The mechanism is uncertain, however.

121 (a) **False**   The incidence of complications tends to be greater after intrathecal administration.

(b) **True**

(c) **False**   These may occur at any dose by all routes.

(d) **True**   Rapid onset of effect causes this.

(e) **False**   Good analgesia has been produced by morphine intrathecally, the disadvantage being the high incidence of side-effects.

122 (a) **True**

(b) **False**

(c) **True**   This is reflected in a larger volume of distribution.

(d) **False**   The pKa of fentanyl is 8.4 compared with 6.5 for alfentanil. Less than 10 per cent of fentanyl is thus unionized at pH of 7.4. This is more than balanced by its high lipid solubility.

(e) **False**   It is much larger.

123 (a) **False**   It is just faster in onset.

(b) **False**

(c) **True**   In fact alfentanil is a useful agent to study this problem.

(d) **True**   There is some suggestion to this effect.

(e) **False**

124 (a) **False**   Sufentanil is about nine times more potent.

(b) **False**   It is similar.

(c) **True**   The concentration of drug at the site of action is more important than the plasma concentration of the drug. Alfentanil, because of its physical properties (Pka, volume of distribution and lipophilic characteristics), has a more rapid onset than sufentanil even though it is less potent.

(d) **True**

(e) **False**   Although there is some uncertainty about the terminal elimination half-life, sufentanil has a larger distribution half-life but a shorter elimination half-life. It is not only the half-lives of alfentanil, sufentanil and fentanyl that are important for determination of recovery but also the size of the compartments into which the drugs redistribute.

125 Naloxone:
    (a) Is most active at mu receptors.
    (b) Has an elimination half-life which is similar to most commonly used opioid drugs.
    (c) Is an effective antagonist of buprenorphine-induced respiratory depression.
    (d) Has no adverse effects other than reversal of analgesia.
    (e) Reverses respiratory depression from inhalational anaesthetic agents.

126 In chronic pain:
    (a) Morphine is useful in the treatment of causalgia.
    (b) Carbamazepine is useful in the treatment of trigeminal neuralgia.
    (c) Streptomycin is useful in the treatment of trigeminal neuralgia.
    (d) Nifedipine is useful in the treatment of reflex sympathetic dystrophy.
    (e) Amitriptyline is useful in the treatment of neuralgia.

127 In migraine:
    (a) The use of beta-adrenergic receptor antagonists is of no benefit.
    (b) Methysergide may carry the risk of retroperitoneal fibrosis.
    (c) Reserpine treatment decreases the incidence of attacks.
    (d) Pizotifen is used prophylactically for aborting an attack.
    (e) Ergot compounds tend to exacerbate an attack.

125 (a) **True** The effects are less at other receptors.

   (b) **False** The elimination half-life of naloxone is considerably shorter than that of most opioids with the possible exception of alfentanil. This is the reason for the reappearance of effects such as respiratory depression when a single dose of naloxone may have been administered in an attempt to counter the effects of high doses of opioids.

   (c) **False** Buprenorphine is a mixed agonist–antagonist drug with affinity for kappa receptors and partial affinity for the mu receptor. Kappa receptors like mu receptors may also mediate respiratory depression. There are suggestions that there are up to four sub-types of kappa receptors, one of which can be found in human placental tissue. Is this the cause of the elevated pain thresholds found in late pregnancy?

   (d) **False** The routine use of naloxone may cause vomiting, diuresis, hypertension, ventricular arrhythmias and even acute pulmonary oedema.

   (e) **False**

126 (a) **False** This severe burning type of pain is associated with injury to peripheral nerves and some degree of sympathetic overactivity.

   (b) **True**

   (c) **True** So called 'wide dynamic range cells' in the dorsal horn of the spinal cord become sensitized so that even normal proprioceptive impulses are interpreted as pain. The mechanism of action of aminoglycosides here is not clear.

   (d) **True** In common with the aminoglycosides, which can have a calcium antagonist-like action.

   (e) **True** This condition can give rise to wide spread pain linked to sensory or autonomic disturbances and drugs with powerful central effects such as amitriptyline may help.

127 (a) **False** Both beta-adrenergic antagonists and calcium entry blockers have been found to be useful in prophylaxis.

   (b) **True**

   (c) **False** Reserpine depletes serotonin (5HT), whose functional deficiency at the $5HT_1$ receptor may have a role in the causation of migraine.

   (d) **True** It is a 5HT antagonist acting at the $5HT_2$ receptors.

   (e) **False** These serotonin agonist drugs remain important for the symptomatic therapy of migraine. There are several types of 5HT receptors. Whereas $5HT_1$ agonists are useful for halting an existing attack, $5HT_2$ antagonists such as methysergide are useful in inhibiting the initial vasoconstriction associated with the onset of migraine, and are therefore used in prophylaxis. $5HT_3$ receptor antagonists such as ondansetron are useful in the treatment of emesis from chemotherapy.

128 Aspirin:
   (a) Induces a tendency to bleeding after the usual therapeutic doses because of inhibition of activated coagulation factors.
   (b) Has a long plasma half-life.
   (c) In overdose leads to hypokalaemic alkalosis.
   (d) In overdose may lead to metabolic acidosis.
   (e) Overdose may be associated with hyperglycaemia in adults.

129 Benorylate:
   (a) Is a prodrug of paracetamol.
   (b) Is unlikely to cause gastric bleeding.
   (c) Unlike aspirin does not potentiate the effects of other anticoagulants.
   (d) Has only central anti-inflammatory properties.
   (e) May cause tinnitus in overdose.

130 Phenylbutazone:
   (a) Is the treatment of choice for inflammatory joint disorders.
   (b) Causes a selective loss of chloride ions and water from the renal tubules.
   (c) Is associated with jaundice.
   (d) Increases the plasma clearance of the active isomer of warfarin.
   (e) Administration may lead to agranulocytosis.

131 Nefopam:
   (a) Is related to orphenadrine.
   (b) Is a potent non-steroidal anti-inflammatory agent.
   (c) Causes marked gastric irritation.
   (d) Does not usually cause respiratory depression.
   (e) Can be safely administered concurrently with monoamine oxidase inhibitors.

132 Sodium salicylate:
   (a) Is an effective inhibitor of prostaglandin synthesis.
   (b) Administration leads to a prolongation of bleeding time.
   (c) Is a less effective analgesic than acetylsalicylic acid
   (d) Is the agent of choice in treating the symptoms of acute rheumatic fever.
   (e) Has respiratory stimulant properties.

128 (a) **False** The mechanism in interference with platelet function.
(b) **False** It is only 15–20 minutes.
(c) **True** This results from vomiting.
(d) **True** This follows the phase of alkalosis.
(e) **True** Hypoglycaemia may occur in children, however. In addition there is hyperpyrexia and dehydration because of stimulant effects on metabolism. Inhibition of succinic dehydrogenase will inhibit the Krebs cycle leading to a ketoacidotic picture particularly in children.

129 (a) **True** It is the acetylsalicylic ester of paracetamol.
(b) **True**
(c) **False** It is no different from aspirin in this respect.
(d) **False** The acetylsalicylic acid content gives it peripheral anti- inflammatory properties.
(e) **True** Aspirin has the same effect.

130 (a) **False** It is not the treatment of choice because of the frequency of side-effects.
(b) **False** Fluid and electrolyte retention and oedema may occur.
(c) **True** Hepatitis could occur.
(d) **False** It is decreased. In addition it displaces warfarin from binding to plasma proteins.
(e) **True**

131 (a) **True**
(b) **False** It is not a non-steroidal anti-inflammatory agent.
(c) **False**
(d) **True** It may give rise to anticholinergic side-effects, however, for example urinary retention and dry mouth.
(e) **False** The analgesic activity of nefopam may be related to monoamine activation in the reticular formation, to control descending inhibitory pathways.

132 (a) **False** Although therapeutic actions of salicylates undoubtedly involve inhibition of prostaglandin biosynthesis, sodium salicylate is an exception. It shares the analgesic properties of aspirin, albeit to a lesser extent, but it does not inhibit prostaglandin synthesis in cell preparations at therapeutic concentrations, nor does it inhibit platelet function significantly. These drugs may also affect neutrophil aggregation by binding to key regulatory proteins in the cell membrane.
(b) **False** For the same reason as above.
(c) **True** The acetylsalicylate ion is more effective than the salicylate ion. However, most of the dose of acetylsalicylic acid is converted to salicylate during first-pass hepatic metabolism.
(d) **False** Sodium salicylate entails too large a sodium load at the doses required for effective treatment.
(e) **True** This is one of the actions of the salicylates that can increase respiratory rate by central stimulation and in overdose by uncoupling oxidative phosphorylation.

133 Paracetamol:
   (a) Has poor anti-inflammatory properties.
   (b) Tends to induce methaemoglobinaemia less frequently than phenacetin.
   (c) Dosage over 20 g in an average adult usually results in death.
   (d) Overdose may be treated with oral methionine.
   (e) Is mainly nephrotoxic when given in an overdose.

134 Diclofenac:
   (a) Is a phenylacetic acid derivative.
   (b) Is a useful analgesic for the treatment of ureteric colic.
   (c) Amongst non-steroidal analgesics is uniquely free from gastrointestinal side-effects.
   (d) Is indicated for the treatment of acute gout.
   (e) Unlike aspirin has no effect on platelet function.

135 Relief from acute gout will be aided by:
   (a) 600 mg aspirin.
   (b) 100 mg allopurinol.
   (c) 100 mg indomethacin.
   (d) 1 mg colchicine.
   (e) Sodium bicarbonate.

136 Ketorolac:
   (a) Is as efficacious as pethidine in mild to moderate pain.
   (b) Has greater analgesic than anti-inflammatory activity.
   (c) Is several hundred times more potent as an analgesic than aspirin.
   (d) Administration results in a prolongation of prothrombin time.
   (e) Does not cause gastric mucosal erosions when given intramuscularly.

133 (a) **True**   Its analgesic effects may depend on inhibition of cyclo-oxygenase in the brain alone.

    (b) **True**

    (c) **True**   Severe hepatotoxicity may result from as little as 10 g. Inadvertent overdosage can easily occur as paracetamol is contained in many brand name 'cold cures'.

    (d) **True**   Conjugation of paracetamol with glucuronide and sulphide in the liver is overwhelmed in paracetamol overdose because of depletion of liver glutathione (whose precursor is methionine) stores, allowing reactive metabolites to produce hepatocellular damage. Damage is worse in alcoholics whose glutathione stores are already depleted. A more common treatment is the infusion of N-acetylcysteine, which is hydrolysed to cysteine (another precursor of glutathione).

    (e) **False**   (See above.)

134 (a) **True**

    (b) **True**   Not only because it is an analgesic but also because it can produce a prolonged fall in urinary output so reducing pressure in an obstructed ureter. The reduction in urinary output comes from the inhibition of renal prostaglandin synthesis. Renal dysfunction may result, however.

    (c) **False**   Gastrointestinal side-effects are common, even ulceration and intestinal perforation have been observed.

    (d) **True**

    (e) **False**   Nevertheless, it has not been shown to produce a significant effect on blood loss in surgery, using the model of transurethral prostatectomy.

135 (a) **False**   Low doses of aspirin encourage uric acid retention, high doses will encourage uric acid loss in the urine but of course are much more likely to cause toxicity. Aspirin is better avoided.

    (b) **False**   This is of no benefit in an acute attack, it may even make matters worse.

    (c) **True**   Its analgesic and anti-inflammatory actions are potent.

    (d) **True**   This works by inhibiting leucocyte migration to the site of urate crystals.

    (e) **True**   As an ancillary measure, urate excretion is increased in alkaline urine.

136 (a) **True**   Also, it does not cause respiratory depression or withdrawal symptoms although a minor degree of sedation may be observed.

    (b) **True**

    (c) **True**

    (d) **False**   It has the anti-platelet effects associated with non-steroidal anti-inflammatory drugs (NSAIDs).

    (e) **False**   It will, of course, induce gastric erosions like other NSAIDs.

137 Lignocaine:
   (a) Is a tertiary amino-ester compound.
   (b) Is usually prepared as an acid salt.
   (c) Is metabolized to para-aminobenzoic acid.
   (d) Is dependent on its lipid solubility for providing analgesia.
   (e) Has a shorter duration of action than bupivacaine because of its greater protein binding.

138 Lignocaine when used in parturient patients:
   (a) May show products of its breakdown in the urine of neonates for 1–3 days after delivery.
   (b) Undergoes diffusion trapping in the foetus.
   (c) Is taken up into the placenta by a process involving active transport.
   (d) May show increased clearance in patients with pre-eclampsia.
   (e) Has no effect on the foetus.

139 Bupivacaine:
   (a) Is slower than lignocaine in its onset of action because of its higher molecular weight.
   (b) Is four times as potent as etidocaine.
   (c) Has a similar therapeutic ratio to lignocaine.
   (d) Unlike lignocaine does not show tachyphylaxis.
   (e) As the carbonated salt has no advantage over the hydrochloride salt.

140 Ropivacaine:
   (a) Is more likely than prilocaine to show methaemoglobinaemia at doses of less than 200 mg.
   (b) Is longer acting than chloroprocaine.
   (c) Induced extradural block is associated with longer lasting and more intense motor block than bupivacaine.
   (d) Is as potent as lignocaine.
   (e) Is as toxic as bupivacaine in animal studies.

141 Cocaine:
   (a) Is a benzoic acid ester.
   (b) Exhibits the same sedative properties as other local anaesthetics.
   (c) Produces mydriasis when applied topically to the eye.
   (d) Is best used mixed with adrenaline when applied to mucous membranes.
   (e) The maximum safe topical dose is 2.5 mg/kg.

137 (a) **False** It is an amino-amide compound.
   (b) **True** It is a basic compound but formulated as an acid salt.
   (c) **False** The esters are metabolized in this way. It is metabolized to xylidides, which have local anaesthetic activity.
   (d) **True** As a rule of thumb, lipid solubility is closely related to intrinsic analgesic potency.
   (e) **False** It is shorter because of less protein binding.

138 (a) **True**
   (b) **True** Lignocaine having crossed the placenta can become ionized, especially in foetal acidosis, thereby trapping the lignocaine in foetal blood. The foetal–maternal concentration ratio of lignocaine in this situation may even be greater than one.
   (c) **False** It is not an active transport process.
   (d) **False** The clearance is reduced.
   (e) **False** There may be some temporary loss of beat to beat variability in the foetal heart rate, and hypotonia in the neonate may also be caused.

139 (a) **False** Although according to Graham's law the rate of diffusion is proportional to molecular weight, this is not important for local anaesthetics since the molecular weights of most local anaesthetics are within a fairly narrow range. Bupivacaine acts relatively slowly because of its greater protein binding and its higher pKa value resulting in greater ionization at body pH.
   (b) **False** It is only marginally more potent than etidocaine.
   (c) **True** It is four times as potent but also four times as toxic.
   (d) **True** For practical purposes.
   (e) **True** Carbonation improves the onset of some other local anaesthetics but not bupivacaine.

140 (a) **False** Methaemoglobin can be formed from 0-toluidine which is a metabolic end product of prilocaine that can convert haemoglobin into methaemoglobin.
   (b) **True** Chloroprocaine is noted for its short duration of action.
   (c) **False** The converse is true.
   (d) **False** It is more potent than lignocaine and only slightly less potent than bupivacaine.
   (e) **False** It is about half as toxic, particularly on the cardiovascular system.

141 (a) **True**
   (b) **False** It is a well-known central stimulant.
   (c) **True** This may be associated with raised intraocular pressure.
   (d) **False** Cocaine produces enough vasoconstriction by itself; adding adrenaline only increases the probability of cardiac dysrhythmias.
   (e) **False** The maximum safe dose is 80–100 mg in an average adult.

142 Amethocaine:
   (a) As a cream can be as effective as EMLA (eutectic mixture of local anaesthetic).
   (b) Is a local anaesthetic of choice in patients susceptible to malignant hyperpyrexia.
   (c) Is metabolized by plasma cholinesterase.
   (d) Is shorter acting than procaine when used for spinal anaesthesia.
   (e) Is chemically related to para-aminobenzoic acid.

143 Lignocaine:
   (a) Toxicity may manifest as circumoral paraesthesia in the early stages.
   (b) Administration is contraindicated in people with epilepsy.
   (c) Overdose usually results in cardiovascular collapse before central nervous system depression.
   (d) In plasma concentrations of 1–2 μg/ml is likely to cause toxicity.
   (e) Has no analgesic activity when administered intravenously.

144 Cocaine:
   (a) In overdose results in death due to medullary depression.
   (b) Possesses antiemetic properties.
   (c) In small doses results in bradycardia.
   (d) Can result in tissue necrosis.
   (e) Abuse leads to stereotypical compulsive behaviour.

Drugs and the gut

145 Cisapride:
   (a) Increases lower oesophageal sphincter pressure.
   (b) Acts by prevention of hydrolysis of acetylcholine.
   (c) Like metoclopramide does not reverse morphine-induced gastric stasis.
   (d) Has no effect on the rate of production of gastric secretions.
   (e) Has no effect on gastric mucosal cell turnover.

146 Cisapride:
   (a) Is a dopamine antagonist.
   (b) Maintains lower oesophageal sphincter pressure in the presence of atropine.
   (c) Increases the bioavailability of cimetidine.
   (d) Unlike metoclopramide increases large bowel motility.
   (e) Is useful in gastric stasis caused by abnormal motility.

142 (a) **True**   In addition it could be faster in onset and longer in duration of action.

   (b) **True**   Amide-type drugs are generally contraindicated.

   (c) **True**   This occurs slowly.

   (d) **False**   It is longer acting.

   (e) **True**   As is benzocaine.

143 (a) **True**

   (b) **False**   Local anaesthetics in therapeutic doses have actually been used in the treatment of convulsive disorders.

   (c) **False**   Central nervous system effects (depression, convulsions or medullary paralysis) occur first leading to hypoxia and acidosis, which may precipitate cardiac arrest.

   (d) **False**   Concentrations of 2–4 μg/ml are often obtained following epidural analgesia with it. Toxic concentrations are usually above 5 μg/ml .

   (e) **False**   It can be used as a systemic analgesic but the therapeutic range is rather narrow.

144 (a) **True**   Central nervous system stimulation leads to euphoria followed by restlessness, convulsions and coma.

   (b) **False**   It stimulates the vomiting centre.

   (c) **True**   Due to central vagal stimulation, larger doses cause tachycardia and hypertension.

   (d) **True**   The nasal septum of chronic abusers is at risk of perforation.

   (e) **True**

---

145 (a) **True**   A useful effect for anti-reflux treatments.

   (b) **False**   It liberates more acetylcholine in the myenteric plexus.

   (c) **False**   Effectiveness against morphine-induced stasis is one of its advantages over metoclopramide.

   (d) **True**

   (e) **True**

146 (a) **False**   Unlike metoclopramide, cisapride has no antagonist effects on dopamine receptors.

   (b) **False**   Disappointing from an anaesthetic point of view.

   (c) **False**   The bioavailability of cimetidine is decreased although that of cisapride itself is increased.

   (d) **True**

   (e) **True**

147 The following statements are correct:
   (a) 10 ml of mist magnesium trisilicate contains 750 mg of magnesium trisilicate and 750 mg of magnesium carbonate.
   (b) 30 ml of 0.3 M sodium citrate contains sufficient alkali to neutralize 150 ml of gastric juice.
   (c) 20 ml of sodium bicarbonate evolves as much carbon dioxide as 30 ml of sodium citrate.
   (d) Magnesium trisilicate, sodium citrate and sodium bicarbonate are equally effective antacids.
   (e) Magnesium trisilicate has the advantage of a longer duration of action as compared to sodium bicarbonate.

148 Omeprazole:
   (a) Controls intragastric acidity irrespective of the stimulus.
   (b) Accelerates gastric emptying.
   (c) Has no effect on the lower oesophageal sphincter.
   (d) Has too short a duration of action to be clinically useful.
   (e) Decreases the pH but not the volume of gastric secretions.

149 Misoprostol:
   (a) Is currently the longest acting H_2-receptor antagonist available.
   (b) Stimulates bicarbonate secretion in the duodenum.
   (c) Administration may cause diarrhoea as a side-effect.
   (d) Increases the proteolytic activity of gastric secretions.
   (e) Is an abortifacient.

150 Ranitidine:
   (a) Is 15 times more potent than cimetidine on a molar basis.
   (b) Has a half-life similar to that of cimetidine.
   (c) Is less likely than cimetidine to inhibit hepatic microsomal enzyme activity.
   (d) Has no consistent effect on the rate of gastric emptying or lower oesophageal sphincter pressure.
   (e) Unlike cimetidine has significant haemodynamic effects on bolus intravenous administration.

151 Cimetidine:
   (a) Is 20 times less potent than famotidine as an H_2-receptor antagonist.
   (b) Is twice as potent as nizatidine as an H_2-receptor antagonist.
   (c) Like famotidine inhibits gastric pepsin secretion.
   (d) Like nizatidine has significant effects on hepatic oxidative metabolism.
   (e) Unlike famotidine is more likely to result in confusion in the elderly.

152 Tri-potassium di-citrato bismuthate:
   (a) Should be taken with an antacid for the immediate relief of dyspepsia.
   (b) Has activity against *Campylobacter (Helicobacter) pylori*.
   (c) Is especially useful in hyperacidity associated with renal failure.
   (d) Increases gastric mucous production.
   (e) Has no anti-pepsin activity.

147 (a) **False**   10 ml of the mixture contain 500 mg each of sodium bicarbonate, magnesium trisilicate and magnesium carbonate along with peppermint emulsion and chloroform water.
 (b) **True**
 (c) **False**   Sodium citrate evolves no carbon dioxide.
 (d) **False**   The efficacy of magnesium trisilicate is not as good because it does not mix well in the stomach and may undergo a layering effect. In addition the particulate matter in it is unsafe itself if aspirated.
 (e) **True**

148 (a) **True**   It prevents the parietal cells from secreting hydrogen ions, as it acts as a proton pump inhibitor.
 (b) **False**   It is not a prokinetic agent.
 (c) **True**
 (d) **False**   The duration of action is long (about 18 hours) although the half-life is considerably shorter.
 (e) **False**   Decreasing pH means greater acidity.

149 (a) **False**   It is a prostaglandin E_1 derivative and not an H_2-receptor antagonist. In addition its duration of action is not as long.
 (b) **True**
 (c) **True**   Because of decreased intestinal water absorption.
 (d) **False**   It is decreased.
 (e) **True**   Hence contraindicated in pregnancy.

150 (a) **False**   It is five times more potent.
 (b) **True**   About 2 hours.
 (c) **True**
 (d) **True**
 (e) **False**   Cimetidine has been associated with cardiac arrest on the bolus administration of 200–400 mg.

151 (a) **True**
 (b) **False**   Nizatidine is about four times more potent.
 (c) **True**
 (d) **False**   Nizatidine has little such known effects.
 (e) **True**

152 (a) **False**   The action of the drug will be impaired by the antacid.
 (b) **True**   This organism may have a role in peptic ulceration by liberation of ammonia.
 (c) **False**   Bismuth, which is potentially neurotoxic, would accumulate in renal failure.
 (d) **True**
 (e) **False**   It inactivates pepsin.

153 Sucralfate:
   (a) Acts as a partial H_2-receptor antagonist.
   (b) Stimulates the secretion of bicarbonate in the stomach.
   (c) Binds to and inactivates pepsin.
   (d) Activity is enhanced by simultaneous administration of an antacid.
   (e) Therapy is limited by its marked laxative effect.

154 Pirenzepine:
   (a) Results in delayed gastric emptying.
   (b) Selectively blocks the secretion of hydrogen ions.
   (c) Reduces the volume of gastric secretions.
   (d) Reduces the secretion of pepsinogen.
   (e) Has more central effects than hyoscine.

155 Carbenoxolone:
   (a) Accelerates gastric emptying.
   (b) Has no effect on acid gastric secretion.
   (c) Enhances mucous secretion in the stomach.
   (d) Accelerates gastric epithelial cell turnover to enhance healing.
   (e) Therapy may result in hyperkalaemia.

156 Loperamide:
   (a) Is a useful treatment for acute diarrhoea in 2-year-old children.
   (b) Enhances the absorption of water from the gut.
   (c) Functions via receptors in the hypothalamus.
   (d) Is a useful symptomatic treatment in severe colitis.
   (e) Results in hypertonia and bradypnoea in overdose.

157 Mesalazine:
   (a) Is enteric-coated sulphapyridine.
   (b) Is useful in ulcerative colitis mainly because of its local effects.
   (c) Is contraindicated in patients with renal impairment.
   (d) May lead to a reduction in the sperm count.
   (e) Is contraindicated in porphyria.

153 (a) **False** It is an aluminium salt of sucrose octasulphate in which the anions bind to positively charged protein molecules exposed in an ulcer base to form a viscous paste, which adheres to the ulcer crater protecting it from the surrounding gastric juice.
   (b) **True** As does mucous.
   (c) **True** Without inhibiting its secretion.
   (d) **False** Sucralfate requires acid to activate it.
   (e) **False** The incidence of side-effects is low with sucralfate.

154 (a) **True** It is a tricyclic drug, which is a selective anticholinergic agent.
   (b) **False** Anticholinergic agents decrease the secretion of both bicarbonate and hydrogen ions, therefore the acid concentration is not lowered. Mucin and proteolytic enzyme secreting cells, rather than the acid secreting cells, are under greater vagal influence.
   (c) **True**
   (d) **True**
   (e) **False** Because of its low lipid solubility.

155 (a) **False** It has no effect on gastric motility.
   (b) **True**
   (c) **True** It creates a mucosal barrier to diffusion of acid.
   (d) **False** It increases the epithelial cell life span and reduces cell turnover.
   (e) **False** It can cause hypokalaemia and other mineralocorticoid-like effects.

156 (a) **False** Rehydration rather than drugs is the most important treatment for diarrhoea. In addition loperamide is not indicated in young children due to a high incidence of side-effects.
   (b) **True** Because of antiperistaltic action.
   (c) **False** Loperamide acts by action on the opioid receptors in the gut. Extensive metabolism in the gut wall and liver ensures that minimal amounts reach systemic circulation. In general terms the antidiarrhoeal activity of opioids has both central and peripheral components. The central effects are mediated by mu receptor activation while the peripheral effects are mediated by both kappa and mu receptor activation. Activation of delta receptors may also result in an antisecretory action in the intestine.
   (d) **False** It may be associated with an increased incidence of toxic megacolon.
   (e) **True** Naloxone may be useful here provided any dehydration is also treated.

157 (a) **False** Mesalazine is 5-aminosalicylic acid in an enteric coating.
   (b) **True** The enteric coating breaks down at pH values of greater than 7 to deliver the drug to the terminal ileum and colon.
   (c) **True** It is excreted via the kidney as N-acetyl-5-aminosalycylic acid.
   (d) **False** This is a feature of sulphasalazine.
   (e) **False** It is sulphasalazine that is contraindicated in porphyria.

158 Chenodeoxycholic acid:
   (a) Acts by increasing the secretion of cholesterol into the bile.
   (b) Is especially useful in the treatment of radio-opaque gall stones.
   (c) Is an example of a drug absorbed by active transport.
   (d) Functions mostly as an inhibitor of 3-hydroxy-3-methyl-glutaryl-coenzyme A
       reductase.
   (e) Is likely to produce greater incidence of side-effects than ursodeoxycholic
       acid.

159 Abnormalities of taste sensation occur with:
   (a) Penicillamine.
   (b) Captopril
   (c) Lithium
   (d) Levodopa
   (e) Metronidazole.

160 Gamolenic acid:
   (a) Is a rich source of linoleic acid.
   (b) May have a beneficial effect in multiple sclerosis.
   (c) May be of benefit in mastalgia.
   (d) Has the same therapeutic efficacy as hydrocortisone in the treatment of
       eczema but without the side-effects.
   (e) May reduce the incidence of seizures in epileptiform states.

161 In the treatment of nausea and vomiting:
   (a) Metoclopramide 10 mg three times a day is effective against cytotoxic
       drug-induced emesis.
   (b) Ondansetron is useful in cytotoxic drug-induced emesis because of its
       dopamine agonist effects.
   (c) Lorazepam has no therapeutic efficacy.
   (d) Domperidone is associated with a lower incidence of extrapyramidal
       reactions than metoclopramide.
   (e) Dexamethasone has a useful therapeutic effect.

162 Emesis associated with anaesthesia:
   (a) Is classically observed after the use of cyclopropane.
   (b) Is more frequent with etomidate than with thiopentone.
   (c) Is less common with ketamine than thiopentone.
   (d) Is more common in men than women.
   (e) Is more common in the elderly.

158 (a) **False** It reduces cholesterol secretion into the bile by inhibiting cholesterol synthesis to a much greater extent than the synthesis of bile
acids and thus creates conditions favourable for the dissolution
of small cholesterol stones.

(b) **False** They contain calcium and are hard to dissolve.

(c) **True** In the terminal ileum.

(d) **True**

(e) **False** Ursodeoxycholic acid is a hydroxy epimer of chenodeoxycholic
acid. It is relatively free from unwanted side-effects especially
diarrhoea.

159 (a) **True**

(b) **True**

(c) **True**

(d) **True**

(e) **True**

160 (a) **True** It is 88 per cent linoleic acid and only 10 per cent gamolenic
acid.

(b) **True** It may shorten the duration of relapse.

(c) **True** Gamolenic acid is converted to dihomo-y-linolenic acid which
plays a part in the metabolism of PG_1 prostaglandins. These in
turn have anti-inflammatory properties.

(d) **False** Hydrocortisone is far more effective although the incidence of
side-effects may be higher.

(e) **False** It may unmask epileptiform activity.

161 (a) **False** Metoclopramide is effective against this type of emesis only
when used in high doses (up to 10 mg/kg given as a slow
infusion). At these doses it acts as a (serotonin) $5\text{-}HT_3$-receptor
antagonist.

(b) **False** Ondansetron is a selective $5\text{-}HT_3$-receptor antagonist, which is
useful in the therapy of emetic symptoms of chemotherapy.

(c) **False** It is similar to that of metoclopramide.

(d) **True** Domperidone is a dopamine antagonist with relatively lower
penetration across the blood–brain barrier and hence a lower
incidence of extrapyramidal reactions.

(e) **True** This is possibly because of interference with the synthesis of
prostaglandins, which are themselves emetic in man.

162 (a) **True**

(b) **True**

(c) **False**

(d) **False** Not really.

(e) **False** It is found less often in the elderly.

Anticholinergics and anticholinesterases

163 Muscarinic receptors:
 (a) In the iris are stimulated by pilocarpine-producing pupillary dilatation.
 (b) In sympathetic ganglionic cells show selective antagonism with pirenzepine.
 (c) In the heart are non-competitively antagonized by vecuronium.
 (d) In the bronchi are antagonized by ipratropium bromide.
 (e) In the bladder are antagonized by distigmine.

164 Hyoscine:
 (a) Is absorbed to a lesser extent than atropine from the gastrointestinal tract.
 (b) Is not absorbed after transdermal application.
 (c) Administration can result in secondary bradycardia.
 (d) Is free from any effect on the lower oesophageal sphincter.
 (e) Unlike atropine is not contraindicated in patients with wide-angle glaucoma.

165 Glycopyrronium (glycopyrrolate):
 (a) Crosses the placenta to cause foetal tachycardia.
 (b) Has no effect on the lower oesophageal sphincter.
 (c) Is superior to hyoscine in suppressing gastric secretions.
 (d) Is free of pupillary effects.
 (e) Has no anti-emetic properties.

166 Atropine:
 (a) Only affects gastric secretions in doses far greater than those producing tachycardia.
 (b) Is more likely than glycopyrronium to cause arrhythmias during anaesthesia.
 (c) Has no effect on foetal heart rate variability.
 (d) Has a greater bronchodilating effect than hyoscine.
 (e) Is a less effective bronchodilator than glycopyrronium.

167 Atropine:
 (a) Is DL-hyoscyamine.
 (b) May interrupt short-term memory.
 (c) May show exaggerated effects in negroes.
 (d) Sulphate has less marked effects on central nervous system than hyoscine butylbromide.
 (e) Causes vasodilatation due to anticholinergic effect on blood vessels.

163 (a) **False**   Although pilocarpine stimulates the muscarinic receptors in the iris, this results in pupillary constriction.

(b) **True**   Pirenzepine blocks the M_1 muscarinic receptors found in the brain and sympathetic ganglia but not the heart. However, the M_2 and M_3 receptors are unaffected.

(c) **False** M_2 muscarinic receptors are found in the heart, nerve terminals and certain cells in sympathetic ganglia. Vecuronium unlike gallamine has no effect on these receptors except in extremely large doses (70–80 x ED95) when a competitive type increase in heart rate may result.

(d) **True**

(e) **False**   This is a cholinesterase drug which acts indirectly by raising the acetylcholine concentrations at the M_3-receptor sites found in smooth muscle, exocrine glands and the endothelium of blood vessels.

164 (a) **True**

(b) **False**   It is absorbed to a significant extent making it of some use in the prevention of sickness.

(c) **True**   Preceded by an initial increase in heart rate.

(d) **False**   Hyoscine relaxes it.

(e) **False**   In normal doses this is not a problem with either drug although intraocular pressure may occasionally increase in patients with narrow-angle glaucoma.

165 (a) **False**   Glycopyrronium is a quaternary ammonium compound and does not cross the blood–brain or the placental barriers.

(b) **False**   This is a peripheral anticholinergic effect.

(c) **True**

(d) **True**   It does not usually show any effects on the eye.

(e) **True**

166 (a) **True**   Atropine in usual clinical doses is not useful as a prophylaxis against acid aspiration.

(b) **True**

(c) **False**   The beat-to-beat variability is usually abolished.

(d) **True**

(e) **False**   They are equally effective.

167 (a) **True**   The L-isomer being the active one for the antimuscarinic activity.

(b) **True**   As does hyoscine.

(c) **True**

(d) **False**   A quaternary compound such as hyoscine butylbromide does not cross the blood–brain barrier.

(e) **False**   Although flushing may occur with high doses of atropine, this is not an antimuscarinic effect as the peripheral blood vessels lack significant cholinergic innervation. The exact mechanism is unknown.

168 Physostigmine:
- (a) Is completely devoid of action on the neuromuscular junction.
- (b) Like neostigmine does not cross the blood–brain barrier.
- (c) Potentiates the effects of tricyclic antidepressant overdose.
- (d) May be used in the treatment of glaucoma.
- (e) May counteract morphine-induced respiratory depression.

169 Edrophonium:
- (a) Is an oxydiaphoretic acetylcholinesterase inhibitor.
- (b) Is the treatment of choice in a cholinergic crisis.
- (c) Shows similar muscarinic activity to neostigmine in clinically useful doses.
- (d) Has more prejunctional activity than neostigmine.
- (e) Is shorter acting than pyridostigmine.

170 Neostigmine:
- (a) Is a prosthetic acetylcholinesterase inhibitor.
- (b) Produces the same duration of acetylcholinesterase inhibition as pyridostigmine.
- (c) Elimination is not influenced by renal failure.
- (d) Is effective in overcoming any aminoglycoside-induced potentiation of neuromuscular blockade.
- (e) Should not be used to antagonize neuromuscular block in patients with glaucoma.

Drugs and the central nervous system

171 Benzodiazepines:
- (a) Act by binding to GABA receptors.
- (b) May produce muscle relaxation via glycine-like actions in the spinal cord.
- (c) May produce anxiolysis by a glycine-like action at brain stem synapses inhibiting afferent conduction to higher centres.
- (d) May enhance the inhibitory effects of glycine in the limbic system to produce an anticonvulsant action.
- (e) Rarely produce retrograde amnesia.

172 Buspirone hydrocloride:
- (a) Is a non-benzodiazepine anxiolytic acting on limbic GABA receptors.
- (b) Is safe in the presence of monoamine oxidase inhibitors.
- (c) Is a useful sedative free from rapid eye movement (REM) sleep suppression.
- (d) Is of no use in treating the benzodiazepine withdrawal syndrome.
- (e) Has no useful muscle relaxant properties.

168 (a) **False** It has some effect, which has, however, been shown to be inadequate for antagonism of neuromuscular block. In addition it has significant central nervous system effects.

  (b) **False** It can cross the blood–brain barrier unlike neostigmine.

  (c) **False** It may have a limited role in the treatment of tricyclic drug overdose.

  (d) **True**

  (e) **True**

169 (a) **False** It is a prosthetic (reversible competitive) inhibitor of acetylcholine. It gets attached to the anionic site on the enzyme. An oxydiaphoretic agent acts as a substrate for the enzyme but one which takes longer to dissociate.

  (b) **False** It would exacerbate the problem. It may be used as a diagnostic tool in small doses.

  (c) **False** It has less pronounced muscarinic effects.

  (d) **True**

  (e) **True** Pyridostigmine is longer acting.

170 (a) **False** It is an oxydiaphoretic agent getting attached to the enzyme at both the esteratic and the anionic sites.

  (b) **False** Pyridostigmine is less potent but longer acting than neostigmine.

  (c) **False** The elimination is prolonged. This may be of potential advantage in patients with renal dysfunction who have been given muscle relaxants.

  (d) **False** 4-aminopyridine may do this.

  (e) **False** The miosis it causes may be useful.

---

171 (a) **False** GABA is an inhibitory neurotransmitter which has binding sites on a protein involved in regulating chloride channels. Benzodiazepine receptors are on the same macromolecular complex but distinct from the GABA receptor.

  (b) **True** Glycine is the major inhibitory neurotransmitter in the spinal cord.

  (c) **True** Anxiolysis probably results from both GABA- and glycine-mediated inhibition of specific neural pathways in the brain.

  (d) **False** Anticonvulsant action is not related to glycine-like effects.

  (e) **True**

172 (a) **False** Buspirone does not act in the same way as the benzodiazepines; it may enhance the activity of specific noradrenergic, dopaminergic and serotonin (5HT) using pathways. There are three 5-HT receptor subtypes, $5\text{-}HT_1$, $5\text{-}HT_2$ and $5\text{-}HT_3$. The $5\text{-}HT_1$ may have 4 different subgroups, A,B, C and D. Buspirone is a $5\text{-}HT_1A$ receptor agonist.

  (b) **False**

  (c) **False** It lacks the sedative, muscle relaxant and anticonvulsant properties of the benzodiazepines.

  (d) **True** It does not control benzodiazepine withdrawal symptoms.

  (e) **True** (See (c)).

173 Benzodiazepines:
   (a) Are rarely associated with light sensitivity dermatitis.
   (b) May release aggression.
   (c) Decrease appetite.
   (d) That do not undergo oxidative metabolism are preferable in patients with hepatic impairment.
   (e) Have no influence on the potency of volatile anaesthetics.

174 Flumazenil:
   (a) Acts partly by enhancing the clearance of benzodiazepines.
   (b) Is ineffective orally because of poor absorption.
   (c) May, in theory, be useful in managing benzodiazepine withdrawal.
   (d) Has been used to reverse coma caused by degeneration of the thalamic nuclei.
   (e) Is without effect in alcohol intoxication.

175 Diazepam:
   (a) Is highly potent because of being less than 50 per cent protein bound.
   (b) Is a weak enzyme inducer.
   (c) But not oxazepam elimination is unaffected by ageing.
   (d) Undergoes hydroxylation in the liver.
   (e) Withdrawn abruptly may lead to convulsions.

176 Zopiclone:
   (a) Is one of a new class of 1,5-benzodiazepine drugs.
   (b) Is safe in hepatic insufficiency as it is excreted unchanged in the urine.
   (c) Has minimal effects on rapid eye movement (REM) sleep.
   (d) Is recommended as an anticonvulsant.
   (e) Administration may give rise to a bitter taste sensation.

177 Benzodiazepines:
   (a) Cross the placenta readily.
   (b) As a class are free from causing respiratory depression.
   (c) Open chloride channels to depolarize excitatory neurones.
   (d) Show pharmacogenetic variation in metabolism.
   (e) While similar in their duration of action differ markedly in their pharmacokinetics.

178 Midazolam:
   (a) Is twice as potent as diazepam.
   (b) Has an elimination half-life half that of diazepam.
   (c) Is poorly absorbed after intramuscular injection.
   (d) Pharmacokinetics is not affected by renal disease.
   (e) Has a lower lipid solubility than diazepam.

173 (a) **True**
   (b) **True**
   (c) **False**
   (d) **True**   This includes drugs like temazepam, oxazepam, lorazepam and lormetazepam.
   (e) **False**   They reduce the MAC value of volatile agents.

174 (a) **False**   Flumazenil reverses all the effects of the benzodiazepine without changing their bioavailability or their kinetics.
   (b) **False**   flumazenil is absorbed after oral administration but extensive first-pass metabolism reduces bioavailability markedly.
   (c) **True**   Benzodiazepine dependence is probably associated with an allosteric change in the benzodiazepine receptor; flumazenil may 'reset' the receptor for normal function.
   (d) **True**   It is used for the same reason in hepatic encephalopathy.
   (e) **False**   (See (d) above.)

175 (a) **False**   Diazepam is over 95 per cent protein bound.
   (b) **True**
   (c) **False**   The elimination of oxazepam that does not undergo demethylation is unaffected by ageing.
   (d) **True**
   (e) **True**

176 (a) **False**   It is not a benzodiazepine. It is a member of the cyclopyrrolone group of compounds with a high affinity for the central nervous system binding sites of the GABA macromolecular receptor complex.
   (b) **False**   It undergoes metabolism in the liver.
   (c) **True**   So it is claimed.
   (d) **False**
   (e) **True**

177 (a) **True**
   (b) **False**   They are all potential respiratory depressants.
   (c) **False**   Opening chloride channels will hyperpolarize a cell.
   (d) **True**
   (e) **False**   While they differ pharmacokinetically, they also differ in the duration of their clinical effects.

178 (a) **True**
   (b) **False**   It is only about one-tenth.
   (c) **False**   Midazolam is well absorbed.
   (d) **True**
   (e) **False**   The water solubility of midazolam disappears at physiological pH with an alteration in the structure of midazolam.

179 Alprazolam:
    (a) Is free from sedative effects.
    (b) May precipitate mania following its administration.
    (c) Unlike diazepam is as potent an antidepressant as some tricyclics.
    (d) Is less potent than diazepam.
    (e) Withdrawal symptoms can be controlled by diazepam.

180 Chloral hydrate:
    (a) Is an effective hypnotic with no effect on rapid eye movement (REM) sleep.
    (b) Is not free from the risk of dependence.
    (c) Increases tolerance for alcohol by enzyme induction.
    (d) Has antiemetic properties.
    (e) Is a useful sedative in hepatic disease.

181 Chlormethiazole:
    (a) Is a metabolite of chloral hydrate.
    (b) Is an anticonvulsant.
    (c) Is effective orally as it does not undergo any first-pass metabolism.
    (d) Is associated with bronchorrhoea.
    (e) Is associated with tachycardia.

182 Midazolam:
    (a) Is more lipid soluble than diazepam.
    (b) Has no effect on systemic vascular resistance.
    (c) Is devoid of any effects on myocardial contractility.
    (d) Produces amnesia unrelated to sedation.
    (e) Is mostly excreted unchanged in the bile.

183 Flumazenil:
    (a) Takes at least 10–15 minutes to exert its effects by intravenous administration.
    (b) In normal doses will be effective for 1–3 hours.
    (c) Can produce nausea and vomiting in 40 per cent of patients.
    (d) Administration can lead to agitation.
    (e) Administration is associated with marked tachycardia.

184 Nightmares may occur during treatment with:
    (a) Clonidine.
    (b) Propranolol.
    (c) Triamterene.
    (d) Metoclopramide.
    (e) Levodopa.

179 (a) **False**
   (b) **True**
   (c) **True**
   (d) **False** It is ten times more potent than diazepam.
   (e) **False** Alprazolam belongs to a new class of potent benzodiazepines with a tricyclic nitrogen ring giving it marked antidepressant activity. It is not free from addiction potential, indeed it can produce severe withdrawal symptoms, which are not controlled by diazepam.

180 (a) **False** Like most hypnotics it causes rapid eye movement (REM) suppression.
   (b) **True**
   (c) **False** It is not to be an enzyme inducer and will compete with alcohol for the enzyme alcohol dehydrogenase.
   (d) **False** It can cause sickness. It has a bitter taste and is a gastric irritant.
   (e) **False**

181 (a) **False** It is a water-soluble thiazole compound.
   (b) **True**
   (c) **False** It is absorbed rapidly following oral administration, although it does show an extensive first-pass effect. This is relevant in patients with hepatic disease where the bioavailability will be much greater.
   (d) **True**
   (e) **True**

182 (a) **True**
   (b) **False** It is reduced.
   (c) **False** It is depressed.
   (d) **True** Amnesia appears to be a separate phenomenon, related to the possible role of GABA receptors in learning. Patients tend to show tolerance to the sedative but not amnesic effects of benzodiazepines.
   (e) **False** It is metabolized by hydroxylation and subsequent conjugation with glucuronic acid. The hydroxy metabolites may have sedative properties.

183 (a) **False** It usually acts within 1–5 minutes. Orally it may take up to 40 minutes.
   (b) **True** It may thus have to be given by infusion when used in intensive care where benzodiazepines may have been used over a long period of time.
   (c) **False** Only in a small proportion of cases.
   (d) **True**
   (e) **False** Cardiovascular stability is generally maintained.

184 (a) **True**
   (b) **True**
   (c) **False**
   (d) **False**
   (e) **True**

185 L-3,4-dihydroxyphenylalanine:
  (a) Is directly metabolized to noradrenaline by catechol-o-methyl transferase.
  (b) Is effective in phenothiazine and butyrophenone-induced Parkinsonism.
  (c) Is usually safe in the presence of selegiline.
  (d) May induce postural hypotension.
  (e) Is frequently associated with nausea.

186 Levodopa is relatively contraindicated in:
  (a) Wide angle glaucoma.
  (b) Malignant melanoma.
  (c) Schizophrenia.
  (d) Recent myocardial infarction.
  (e) Opiate-induced pruritus.

187 Co-beneldopa:
  (a) Produces a much lower incidence of nausea than levodopa alone.
  (b) Has the same incidence of drug-induced involuntary movements as levodopa alone.
  (c) Treatment is not associated with on–off phenomena.
  (d) Is much more likely to be associated with agitation than levodopa alone.
  (e) Has a greater risk of cardiac arrhythmias than levodopa.

185 (a) **False** L-dihydroxyphenylalanine is levodopa which can cross the blood–brain barrier to be metabolized by dopa-decarboxylase to dopamine and only then to noradrenaline and adrenaline.

   (b) **False** Parkinsonism induced by these drugs is not usually caused by lack of dopamine but blockade of the dopamine receptors.

   (c) **True** Selegiline is an exception among monoamine oxidase inhibitors in this respect and is used in the treatment of this condition.

   (d) **True** Although the mechanism is not clear.

   (e) **True** But this should not be treated with phenothiazines.

186 (a) **False** It should not, however, be used in the presence of narrow-angle glaucoma.

   (b) **True** As it is a precursor of melanin.

   (c) **True** The main dopamine-using neural pathways in the brain are the mesolimbic, the intrahypothalamic and the nigrostriatal. Levodopa acts as an anti-Parkinsonian agent by increasing the dopamine concentrations in the nigrostriatal pathways. However, this also results in increased dopamine concentrations in the mesolimbic pathway, which can facilitate development of psychotic symptoms. This explains the development of Parkinsonism-like side-effects from the use of antidopaminergic agents, such as chlorpromazine, in the treatment of psychotic disorders.

   (d) **True** Although levodopa is principally metabolized to 3,4-dihydroxy-phenylacetic acid and 3-methoxy-4-hydroxyphenylacetic acid small amounts are also converted to noradrenaline and adrenaline, which would be contraindicated in someone with a recent infarct.

   (e) **False**

187 (a) **True** By adding a peripheral dopa decarboxylase inhibitor (benserazide) to levodopa, the overall dose of levodopa can be reduced, resulting in lower side-effects.

   (b) **True** Involuntary movements are a central effect.

   (c) **False** As is the case with levodopa alone.

   (d) **False** It is once again a central effect of dopamine.

   (e) **False** Because the dose of levodopa is smaller.

188 Selegiline:
   (a) Is chemically related to amphetamine.
   (b) Is a reversible monoamine oxidase inhibitor.
   (c) Slows the progression of Parkinson's disease.
   (d) Will attenuate many of the fluctuations of motor function in Parkinson's disease.
   (e) When added to a dose of levodopa will significantly reduce the incidence of confusion and hallucinations or other peak-dose side-effects.

189 Amantadine:
   (a) Acts partly by releasing dopamine by central neurons.
   (b) Is less effective than levodopa.
   (c) Induced improvements in Parkinson's disease are well sustained
   (d) Should not be co-prescribed with levodopa.
   (e) Is of use in Huntington's chorea.

190 Pergolide:
   (a) Decreases levodopa requirements in Parkinson's disease.
   (b) May result in both hypotension and hypertension
   (c) Decreases peripheral levodopa metabolism.
   (d) Tends to reduce the end of dose effects of levodopa.
   (e) May reduce the effectiveness of bromocriptine.

188 (a) **True**   It is L-N-propynyl-methamphetamine. It is metabolized *in vivo* to
                      L-amphetamine and L-methamphetamine, but unlike the corre-
                      sponding dextrorotatory forms there are few adverse effects from
                      these metabolites.

   (b) **False**   It is a fairly selective inhibitor, which binds irreversibly to the
                      isoenzyme monoamino oxidase-B.

   (c) **True**   Patients treated with selegiline may live without levodopa for
                      longer periods. Why this should be the case is not clear.
                      Selegiline may decrease the generation of free radicals in the
                      nigrostriatal pathway or it may prevent the production of some
                      selective nigral toxin. The chemical 1-methyl-4-phenyl-1,2,3,6-
                      tetrahydropyridine (MPTP) can be formed as a by-product of
                      the illegal home manufacture of fentanyl. Addicts using this con-
                      taminated fentanyl developed Parkinsonian symptoms, because
                      MPTP, while not itself toxic, was oxidized by monoamino oxidase-
                      B to a reactive metabolite which damaged mitochondria. This
                      toxicity can be reduced by pretreatment with selegiline.

   (d) **True**   Some patients experience a gradual reduction in their response
                      to levodopa after treatment for some time; it is in these
                      patients that treatment with selegiline restores responsiveness
                      and decreases the 'wearing off' effects of levodopa.

   (e) **False**   Unless the dose is reduced peak-dose side-effects can get worse
                      if selegiline is added; the alternative is to decrease the dose of
                      levodopa before adding selegiline but at the risk of exacerbating
                      Parkinsonian symptoms. A dilemma for the doctor!

189 (a) **True**   Although the precise mode of action is unknown.
   (b) **True**   But more effective than anticholinergic drugs.
   (c) **False**   The effect starts waning after a few months.
   (d) **False**   It may be used to decrease levodopa requirements as well as to
                      improve the 'on–off' effects in Parkinsonism.
   (e) **False**   Levodopa or drugs enhancing the effects of dopamine will
                      exacerbate this condition. As a result dopamine antagonists are
                      used to control symptoms in this condition.

190 (a) **True**   This is a directly acting dopamine agonist with a relatively long
                      duration of action.

   (b) **True**   The drug is active at both dopamine$_1$ and dopamine$_2$ receptors
                      (D_1,D_2) and also has weak alpha$_2$ stimulating properties. It acts
                      primarily at D_2 receptors in the corpus striatum and unlike
                      bromocriptine it does not partially antagonize D_1 receptors.
                      Dopamine D_2 receptor stimulation can mediate hypotension,
                      while at large doses alpha$_2$ stimulation results in vasopressor
                      responses.

   (c) **False**
   (d) **True**   It can suppress fluctuations in the response to levodopa.
   (e) **False**   It is like bromocriptine but with a marginally better therapeutic
                      ratio.

191 Benzhexol:
   (a) Is most effective in the akinesia of Parkinson's disease.
   (b) Is effective in treating tremor.
   (c) Is supplementary to treatment with levodopa.
   (d) Is effective in tardive dyskinesia.
   (e) Is effective in drug-induced dystonic reactions.

192 Tricyclic antidepressants:
   (a) Potentiate membrane pumps liberating 5-hydroxytryptamine, noradrenaline or dopamine.
   (b) May antagonize the effects of reserpine.
   (c) Possess antiepileptic activity.
   (d) Improve psychomotor performance in depressed patients.
   (e) Are associated with diarrhoea.

193 Toxic effects of tricyclic antidepressants may include:
   (a) Weight loss.
   (b) Acute urinary retention.
   (c) Tinnitus.
   (d) Impotence.
   (e) Prolongation of PR interval more commonly than prolongation of the QT interval.

194 Monoamine oxidase inhibitors:
   (a) Can be useful in the treatment of migraine.
   (b) Lead to postural hypotension.
   (c) Are associated with greater hypertensive reactions to directly acting sympathomimetics than indirectly acting agents.
   (d) Act more rapidly than the tricyclic antidepressants in the treatment of endogenous depression.
   (e) Are useful in the treatment of obsessive–compulsive disorders.

195 Carbamazepine:
   (a) Is the drug of first choice in trigeminal neuralgia.
   (b) Is effective against petit mal seizures.
   (c) Shows autoinduction.
   (d) Dosage needs to be increased in patients concurrently receiving diltiazem.
   (e) Is relatively contraindicated in those treated with lithium.

191 (a) **False**   Although antimuscarinic agents have long been used in the treatment of Parkinson's disease because they may compensate for a relative excess of cholinergic activity induced by dopamine deficiency, they are most effective in reducing tremor and not akinesia.

   (b) **True**   (See (a) above.)

   (c) **True**   Whereas levodopa is most effective against akinesia, benzhexol is useful in reducing the rigidity and tremor.

   (d) **False**   It will make this worse. This can be thought of as a hypersensitivity state in the nigrostriatal pathway brought on by chronic dopamine receptor blockade.

   (e) **True**   Although acute reactions are treated with parenterally administered agents such as benztropine.

192 (a) **False**   They block the neuronal re-uptake of these amines.

   (b) **True**

   (c) **False**   They have epileptogenic potential.

   (d) **True**   But not in normal subjects.

   (e) **False**   They have some anticholinergic effects and so may cause constipation.

193 (a) **False**   There may be weight gain.

   (b) **True**   This is an uncommon action linked to their anticholinergic activity.

   (c) **True**   This is rare.

   (d) **True**

   (e) **False**   It is the reverse (about 11 per cent against 86 per cent). Prolonged QT interval is one of the principal mechanisms of provoking arrhythmias.

194 (a) **False**   They often aggravate migraine.

   (b) **True**   Increased alpha stimulation of the vasomotor centre causes a reflex decrease in blood pressure.

   (c) **False**   The interaction is greater with indirect agents.

   (d) **False**   The clinical response may take several weeks to appear.

   (e) **True**   Along with some types of facial pain and endogenous depression.

195 (a) **True**   An established indication for which a pain clinic might use the drug.

   (b) **False**   It is used against grand mal and focal seizures.

   (c) **True**   It is a well known enzyme inducer, which induces its own metabolism.

   (d) **False**   Its plasma levels are actually increased.

   (e) **True**   There is a risk of neurotoxicity despite normal plasma levels.

196 Lithium:
   (a) Is superior to tricyclic drugs because it is effective within 24 hours.
   (b) Toxicity can be precipitated by bendrofluazide.
   (c) Has a wide therapeutic range.
   (d) Is useful in drug-induced diabetes insipidus.
   (e) Therapy may increase the dose requirement of suxamethonium.

197 Drug-induced depression can be a feature of:
   (a) Captopril.
   (b) Verapamil.
   (c) Clonidine
   (d) Alpha-methyldopa.
   (e) Reserpine.

198 Phenothiazine drugs:
   (a) Are selective in the treatment of schizophrenia.
   (b) Decrease prolactin release.
   (c) Are antiemetic because of their effects on the mesolimbic system.
   (d) Have a quinidine-like action on the heart.
   (e) Often induce anorexia.

199 Droperidol:
   (a) Is a potent hypnotic related to the butyrophenones.
   (b) Is the most effective agent in preventing motion sickness.
   (c) May exert a useful antiarrhythmic effect during anaesthesia.
   (d) Is a potent amnesic agent.
   (e) Is not suitable for use in patients with Parkinsonism.

200 Haloperidol:
   (a) Has less potent sedative properties than chlorpromazine.
   (b) Is more likely to produce hypotension than chlorpromazine.
   (c) Is more likely to produce extrapyramidal effects than chlorpromazine.
   (d) Is a less effective antiemetic than chlorpromazine against opiates.
   (e) Should be used with caution in the presence of methyldopa.

196 (a) **False** It may take 10–14 days to exert beneficial effects just like the tricyclic drugs.

(b) **True** Because of decreased renal clearance.

(c) **False**

(d) **False** It is a cause of polydipsia and polyuria possibly via a suppression of antidiuretic hormone activity.

(e) **False** It may potentiate the action of both depolarizing and non-deploarizing relaxants.

197 (a) **False** ACE inhibitors have widespread effects in the body but drug-induced depression is not one of them. It may be associated with the opposite effect when given to treat hypertension in depressed patients.

(b) **False** There is no evidence to this effect.

(c) **False** Although sedative, large studies have failed to show a higher than expected incidence of depression in patients treated with it.

(d) **True** Possibly in a dose-related manner in up to 10 per cent of patients.

(e) **True** In a dose-related manner.

198 (a) **False** They exert beneficial effects in virtually all types of psychotic illnesses.

(b) **False** The release of prolactin is increased because of their anti-dopaminergic activity in the intra-hypothalamic (tubero-infundibular) pathway.

(c) **False** The antiemetic effect is due to action on the chemoreceptor trigger zone.

(d) **True**

(e) **False** Increased appetite and weight gain are common.

199 (a) **False** It is not a potent hypnotic. Used alone it leads to apparent outward tranquillity which, in fact, is associated with mental anguish.

(b) **False** It is a powerful antiemetic, most effective against the opioid-induced emesis. Hyoscine is more effective against motion sickness.

(c) **True** This is useful during dental surgery.

(d) **False**

(e) **True** Because of its antidopaminergic effects.

200 (a) **True** But as with droperidol it may produce an outwardly calm appearance.

(b) **False** Its alpha receptor blocking activity is weak.

(c) **True** In addition it is longer acting.

(d) **False** It is more potent because of its greater anti-dopaminergic action.

(e) **True** Because of additional sedative effect of methyldopa and the possibility of mental disturbances.

201 Chlorpromazine:
   (a) Is structurally similar to gamma-aminobutyric acid.
   (b) Produces a profound fall in basal metabolic rate.
   (c) Is associated with menorrhagia.
   (d) Exerts a strong antihistaminic effect.
   (e) Is associated with postural hypotension.

202 Among phenothiazines:
   (a) Those with a piperazine side chain are powerful anti-psychotic drugs.
   (b) Those with an aliphatic side chain exhibit alpha-adrenergic receptor blocking effects.
   (c) Those with a piperidine side chain are more likely to produce extrapyramidal reactions.
   (d) Those with a piperazine side chain are less likely to produce sedation.
   (e) Those with an aliphatic side chain are least likely to produce extrapyramidal reactions.

203 Clozapine:
   (a) May be effective when other neuroleptics fail.
   (b) Has a low risk of tardive dyskinesia.
   (c) Has a high risk of extrapyramidal symptoms.
   (d) Can lead to agranulocytosis.
   (e) Can be administered to nursing mothers.

204 Clomipramine:
   (a) Is useful in the treatment of obsessive compulsive disorders.
   (b) Is the most potent serotonin re-uptake inhibitor among the tricyclic anti-depressants.
   (c) Has troublesome anticholinergic side-effects.
   (d) Can lead to postural hypotension.
   (e) Has a lower fatal toxicity index than other tricyclics drugs.

205 Mianserin:
   (a) Is an atypical tricyclic antidepressant.
   (b) Acts presynaptically to increase amine synthesis.
   (c) Is less effective in younger patients.
   (d) Results in fewer antimuscarinic side-effects than the typical tricyclic antidepressants.
   (e) Can result in blood dyscrasias in about one in 5000 patients.

201 (a) **True**   It contains a propylene chain terminating in a tertiary nitrogen atom, which is a common structural property of neuroleptic agents.

   (b) **False**   It has little effect on the metabolic rate although it interferes with thermoregulation by inhibiting hypothalamic function.

   (c) **False**   It increases prolactin release producing galactorrhoea and amenorrhoea.

   (d) **False**   Its antihistaminic effect is weak.

   (e) **True**

202 (a) **True**   Such as fluphenazine and trifluoperazine.

   (b) **True**

   (c) **False**   It is more common in drugs with a piperazine chain.

   (d) **True**

   (e) **False**   The aliphatic side chain compounds, represented by chlorpromazine, exhibit powerful anti-psychotic, moderate alpha receptor blocking and moderate extrapyramidal activity. The piperazine group represented by prochloroperazine is the most likely and the piperadine group, represented by thioridazine, is the least likely group producing extrapyramidal reactions. A potential problem with the piperidine side chain drugs is the risk of damage to the eye.

203 (a) **True**   It is indicated for schizophrenia when patients have failed to respond to conventional drugs. It is a dibenzodiazepine as opposed to being a phenothiazine. It is unusual in that it may not chronically alter D_2-receptor function in the nigrostriatal pathway, thus being associated with a lower risk of tardive dyskinesia.

   (b) **True**

   (c) **False**

   (d) **True**   Regular checks on the white cell count must be made.

   (e) **False**   It is excreted in breast milk.

204 (a) **True**

   (b) **True**   It is not clear if this is the reason for its superiority over other tricyclic agents in the treatment of compulsive disorders.

   (c) **True**   Dry mouth, sweating, blurred vision and constipation are common.

   (d) **True**   Probably the most frequent of the cardiovascular side-effects caused by this drug.

   (e) **True**   The fatal toxicity index is the number of deaths per million prescriptions and is lower with this drug; nevertheless deaths after overdose can still occur.

205 (a) **False**   It is not a tricyclic agent.

   (b) **True**   In contrast to the tricyclics, which are inhibitors of transmitter amine re-uptake.

   (c) **False**   There is no evidence for this.

   (d) **True**   Postural hypotension is also less marked.

   (e) **True**   More so in the elderly.

206 Among the tricyclic drugs, amitryptiline:
   (a) Is the most sedative.
   (b) Is unique in having no active metabolites.
   (c) Is more likely to be associated with postural hypotension.
   (d) Has the least antimuscarinic effects.
   (e) Is not likely to be associated with arrhythmias under anaesthesia.

207 Phenelzine:
   (a) Has less side-effects than tranylcypromine.
   (b) Toxicity is influenced by acetylator phenotype.
   (c) May result in urinary incontinence.
   (d) Frequently results in addiction.
   (e) Can result in withdrawal symptoms.

208 Phenytoin:
   (a) Raises the seizure threshold in the brain.
   (b) Is free from sedation at normal doses.
   (c) Shows excellent intramuscular absorption.
   (d) Shows considerable pharmacogenetic variation in its metabolism.
   (e) Shows non-linear kinetics.

209 Phenytoin toxicity:
   (a) Is more likely in the presence of sulphonamides.
   (b) Is more likely in the presence of carbamazepine.
   (c) May manifest itself as megaloblastic anaemia.
   (d) May manifest itself as seizures.
   (e) May manifest itself as nystagmus.

210 Sodium valproate:
   (a) Inhibits the effects of gamma aminobutyric acid in the brain.
   (b) Shows good correlation between plasma concentrations and effect.
   (c) Is particularly effective in the treatment of absence seizures.
   (d) Can result in fulminant hepatitis.
   (e) May be associated with bleeding after major surgery.

211 Ethosuximide:
   (a) Is particularly effective in the management of childhood tonic seizures.
   (b) Should not be co-administered with phenytoin.
   (c) May lead to a systemic lupus erythematosus-like syndrome.
   (d) May result in pancytopenia.
   (e) Has the advantage of being free from any gastrointestinal side-effects.

206 (a) **True**   At the other end of the spectrum is protriptyline that may have a stimulant action.
  (b) **False**   Nortriptyline is an active metabolite although less sedating.
  (c) **True**   Whereas doxepin, for example, is less active in this regard.
  (d) **False**   Along with imipramine it has considerable antimuscarinic effects.
  (e) **False**   Especially in the presence of halothane.

207 (a) **True**
  (b) **True**
  (c) **False**   Urinary retention may occur due to its antimuscarinic effects.
  (d) **False**   This is seen most often with tranylcypromine.
  (e) **True**   Headache, shivering, paraesthesia and nightmares may result within days of withdrawing the drug. These are symptoms of withdrawal after addiction and not a return of the depressive illness.

208 (a) **False**   It stops the spread of the seizure process without apparently affecting the seizure threshold.
  (b) **True**
  (c) **False**   Intramuscular administration can result in the drug crystallizing in the tissues.
  (d) **True**   There are slow and fast metabolizers.
  (e) **True**

209 (a) **True**   Because phenytoin is 90 per cent protein bound to albumin and alpha-globulins, from which it may be displaced.
  (b) **False**   The metabolism of phenytoin is increased.
  (c) **True**   This responds to folate administration.
  (d) **True**   A paradoxical increase in the number of seizures.
  (e) **True**   A fairly early sign.

210 (a) **False**   It potentiates the effects of GABA. At 'supra-clinical' doses it can even inhibit enzymes involved in the degradation of GABA.
  (b) **False**   The correlation is relatively poor.
  (c) **True**
  (d) **True**   This is rare but worrying, and is found especially in children under 3 years of age.
  (e) **True**   This is an effect on the second stage of platelet aggregation or rarely because of thrombocytopenia.

211 (a) **False**   It is a drug of choice in absence seizures.
  (b) **False**   It can be used in combination.
  (c) **True**   Along with a variety of rashes.
  (d) **True**
  (e) **False**   These and the central nervous system side-effects are frequent with this drug.

212 Ethanol:
  (a) Is useful in the treatment of methanol poisoning.
  (b) Is excreted in the urine to an extent of 45 per cent.
  (c) Is found in expired air in a concentration of about 0.05 per cent of that in the blood.
  (d) Potentiates the effects of gamma-aminobutyric acid.
  (e) Is unlikely to produce unconsciousness at blood concentration of 300 mg/dl.

213 Paroxetine:
  (a) Is a serotonin ($5HT_{1A}$) agonist.
  (b) Is effective in depression combined with anxiety.
  (c) May exacerbate mania.
  (d) Can safely be administered along with phenytoin without the risk of side-effects.
  (e) Has nausea as its most common adverse effect.

214 Phencyclidine administration:
  (a) May lead to an acute confusional state.
  (b) Can be associated with unpredictable violent behaviour.
  (c) Is associated with nystagmus.
  (d) Is associated with analgesia.
  (e) Is associated with gross ataxia.

Antimicrobial and immunosuppressant drugs

215 The mode of action of:
  (a) Chloramphenicol is to block bacterial protein synthesis.
  (b) Cefamandole is to prevent messenger RNA synthesis.
  (c) Ciprofloxacin is to inhibit bacterial DNA gyrase.
  (d) Benzylpenicillin is to prevent the replication of bacterial DNA.
  (e) Metronidazole is to inhibit dihydrofolate reductase metabolism.

212 (a) **True**   Methanol is metabolized by alcohol dehydrogenase to formic acid, which is responsible for the toxicity. This can be reduced by administering ethanol, which competes as substrate for the enzyme.

   (b) **False**   The urinary concentration of ethanol may be about 130 per cent of the blood concentration even though over 90 per cent of ethanol is metabolized in the liver.

   (c) **True**

   (d) **True**   By interacting with the GABA-benzodiazepine-chloride ionophore.

   (e) **False**   Ethanol at concentrations of about 100 mg/dl produces impairment of mental function and slurred speech, at 200 mg/dl many people will be unresponsive, at 300 mg/dl most will be comatose and levels of 500 mg/dl may be fatal. In addition it is important to remember that ethanol and other cerebral depressants may have additive or potentiating effects thus requiring lower concentrations to produce unconsciousness.

213 (a) **False**   It is a serotonin re-uptake inhibitor like fluoxetine, sertaline and fluvoxamine. They may have a better side-effect profile than ordinary tricyclic antidepressants possibly resulting in better compliance.

   (b) **True**   Perhaps this is a feature of drugs enhancing the action of serotonin.

   (c) **True**

   (d) **False**   The incidence of side-effects is higher in the presence of phenytoin.

   (e) **True**   This is a feature of typical serotonin re-uptake inhibitors. In addition these agents often cause loss of appetite.

214 (a) **True**   Phencyclidine in powder form is also known as 'angel dust'!
   (b) **True**
   (c) **True**
   (d) **True**
   (e) **True**

---

215 (a) **True**   By binding to bacterial ribosomes and inhibiting peptidyl-transferase to block protein synthesis.

   (b) **False**   It acts almost the same way as benzylpenicillin (see (d) below).

   (c) **True**

   (d) **False**   It belongs to the beta-lactam ring group of antibiotics whose action is to interfere with bacterial cell wall synthesis. Penicillins and cephalosporins are structurally similar to peptidoglycan polymers which make up the bacterial cell wall and so can compete with enzymes that catalyse cross-linking of these polymers.

   (e) **False**   It penetrates into the anaerobic bacteria where its hydroxylamine derivative inhibits DNA replication, transcription and repair.

216 Sulphonamides:
  (a) As a group have a similar spectrum of activity.
  (b) Are bactericidal.
  (c) That are applied topically are more likely to be associated with the Stevens–Johnson syndrome.
  (d) May produce kernicterus.
  (e) Are mainly used for uncomplicated urinary tract infections.

217 Cefamandole:
  (a) Has a broad spectrum of activity against both Gram-positive and Gram-negative organisms.
  (b) May show enhanced nephrotoxicity in the presence of diuretics.
  (c) May show an antabuse-type reaction with alcohol.
  (d) Enhances the action of warfarin.
  (e) Can be associated with neutropenia.

218 Cyclosporin:
  (a) Is a cephalosporin with very low antibiotic activity.
  (b) Has its main site of action within T lymphocytes.
  (c) Is particularly effective in ocular manifestations of Behcet's disease.
  (d) Can give rise to alopecia.
  (e) Is associated with irreparable renal damage.

219 Erythromycin:
  (a) Acts by inhibition of bacterial cell wall formation.
  (b) Administration may result in hearing loss.
  (c) Can be associated with haemolytic jaundice.
  (d) Potentiates the action of warfarin.
  (e) Should preferably be administered by infusion in acute infections.

220 Netilmicin:
  (a) Is highly active against Gram-negative bacilli.
  (b) Frequently shows synergism with cephalosporins in the treatment of *Pseudomonas* infections.
  (c) Is less nephrotoxic than gentamicin.
  (d) Is more nephrotoxic than amikacin.
  (e) Has much the same toxic effect on vestibular function as streptomycin.

216 (a) **True**
    (b) **False**   They are bacteriostatic.
    (c) **False**   Stevens–Johnson syndrome is linked to long-acting highly protein-bound agents.
    (d) **True**   By displacing bilirubin from protein binding sites.
    (e) **True**

217 (a) **True**   With the exception of *Pseudomonas*.
    (b) **True**   And also in the presence of aminoglycosides.
    (c) **True**   As it inhibits acetaldehyde dehydrogenase. This may be important if a parenteral feeding regimen contains alcohol.
    (d) **True**   And it can rarely cause thrombocytopenia by itself.
    (e) **True**   Usually after a long course of administration.

218 (a) **False**   It is lipophilic cyclic undecapeptide isolated from the fungus *Tolypocladium inflatum gams* and is an immunosuppressant.
    (b) **True**   It binds to cyclophilin, a cytosolic protein, leading to alterations in the lymphocyte that impede the transcription of lymphokine genes and inhibit the release of interleukin-2 and other growth factors for lymphocytes. This creates a temporary immune paralysis.
    (c) **True**   Cyclosporin has been assessed with varying degrees of success in a variety of transplant operations and autoimmune disorders. It has also shown promise in myasthenia gravis, rheumatoid arthritis and even Crohn's disease.
    (d) **False**   It can cause hypertrichosis.
    (e) **True**   Cyclosporin in high doses can produce changes which progress to interstitial fibrosis of the kidney.

219 (a) **False**   It inhibits protein synthesis from bacterial ribosomes but not human ones.
    (b) **True**   But it is transient and reversible.
    (c) **False**   Cholestatic jaundice can occur with erythromycin estolate; it is reversible.
    (d) **True**   As also of digoxin, carbamazepine and theophylline.
    (e) **True**   Because of damage to the veins.

220 (a) **True**
    (b) **True**   This is a commonly used combination but also carries a greater risk of nephrotoxicity.
    (c) **True**
    (d) **False**
    (e) **False**   Netilmicin tends to damage the auditory component of the eighth nerve.

221 The spectrum of antimicrobial activity of:
   (a) Amoxycillin plus clavulanic acid includes *Haemophilus influenzae*.
   (b) Mezlocillin makes it the most active of the acylureido penicillins against *Pseudomonas aeruginosa*.
   (c) Cloxacillin includes *Staphylococcus aureus*.
   (d) Mecillinam includes *Pseudomonas aeruginosa*.
   (e) Bacampicillin includes *Listeria monocytogenes*.

222 Mupirocin:
   (a) Is the drug of choice for the treatment of *E. Coli* septicaemia.
   (b) Inhibits bacterial cell wall formation.
   (c) Is effective by topical application in impetigo.
   (d) Is effective against methicillin-resistant strains of *Staphylcoccus aureus*.
   (e) Therapy may cause ototoxicity.

223 Teicoplanin:
   (a) Acts by interfering with the bacterial DNA synthesis.
   (b) Is mostly indicated in the treatment of Gram-positive infections.
   (c) Therapy is limited by its short duration of action.
   (d) Is just as likely as vancomycin to produce the 'Red Man' syndrome.
   (e) Unlike the aminoglycosides is not associated with ototoxicity.

224 Imipenem:
   (a) Is limited to activity against *Listeria monocytogenes*.
   (b) Requires the co-administration of cilastatin to be effective against *Haemophilus influenzae*.
   (c) Is free from the risk of *Pseudomembranous colitis*.
   (d) Is nephrotoxic in animals but much less so in man.
   (e) Administration may result in red urine.

221 (a) **True** The addition of clavulanic acid, a bacterial beta-lactamase inhibitor, extends the antibacterial spectrum of amoxycillin to *Haemophilus* and many of the enterobacteriaceae.

 (b) **False** Azlocillin is the most active of this group with 2–4 times the activity of ticarcillin or mezlocillin.

 (c) **True**

 (d) **False** It has considerable activity against many Gram-negative bacteria but not *Pseudomonas*.

 (e) **True** Although this is just an ester of ampicillin which is better absorbed from the gut.

222 (a) **False** This drug is used only by topical application.

 (b) **False** It has a novel mode of action inhibiting bacterial protein synthesis by competitively blocking isoleucyl transfer-RNA synthesis.

 (c) **True**

 (d) **True** This is the main indication for the drug. It can be used as a nasal cream to treat carriers of methicillin-resistant *Staphylococci* which has become a problem in several hospitals around the world.

 (e) **False** What little of the drug that is absorbed is metabolized without toxic effects.

223 (a) **False** It inhibits peptidoglycan elongation thus preventing cell wall synthesis mostly in Gram-positive organisms. Gram-negative organisms have an external lipid membrane which prevents a large molecule like teicoplanin from reaching the peptidoglycan layer.

 (b) **True**

 (c) **False** Its duration of action is long enough, therefore it only needs to be administered once a day.

 (d) **False** The 'Red Man' syndrome in which there is pruritus, erythema, angioedema and profound hypotension sometimes occurs after administration of vancomycin and is due to histamine release. Teicoplanin is considered a safer and a more convenient alternative to vancomycin.

 (e) **False** It has been linked to ototoxicity but not as often.

224 (a) **False** It has a broad spectrum of activity although it is not indicated for central nervous system infections.

 (b) **False** It is active by itself. However cilastatin increases the urinary tract concentration of imipenem by reversibly inhibiting dehydropeptidase I, an enzyme of the renal tubular brush border, which is involved in the metabolism of imipenem. The nephrotoxicity of imipenem may also be reduced even further.

 (c) **False**

 (d) **True** (See (b) above.)

 (e) **True** It is red urine not haematuria, particularly in children.

225 Ciprofloxacin:
  (a) Is of little value against Gram-negative organisms.
  (b) Is preferentially concentrated in the lungs.
  (c) Increases the requirements of theophylline by inducing its metabolism.
  (d) Is relatively contraindicated at times of growth.
  (e) Is not absorbed after oral administration.

226 Treatment with:
  (a) Acyclovir is indicated in *Herpes simplex* encephalitis.
  (b) Ganciclovir is of no therapeutic value in life-threatening cytomegalovirus infection.
  (c) Tribavirin is indicated in severe respiratory syncytial virus bronchiolitis.
  (d) Inosine pranobex is indicated in *Herpes simplex*.
  (e) Zidovudine is indicated in *Herpes simplex*.

227 Zidovudine:
  (a) Acts by preventing human immunodeficiency virus (HIV) from uncoating its RNA in the host cells.
  (b) Is best administered once a day.
  (c) Therapy may become ineffective due to development of resistance after treatment for 6 months or more.
  (d) Is particularly effective against HIV-induced neutropenia.
  (e) May show an increased incidence of adverse effects if co-administered with paracetamol.

228 Acyclovir:
  (a) Unlike zidovudine, cannot be administered on a long-term basis to control recurrent infection in the immunocompromised subject.
  (b) Unlike ganciclovir, has little effect on bone marrow in therapeutic doses.
  (c) Unlike ganciclovir, is associated with convulsions if co-administered with imipenem.
  (d) Is superior to inosine pranobex in the treatment of primary genital herpes.
  (e) Cannot be co-administered with interferon alpha-2a.

229 Bleomycin:
  (a) Is metabolized extensively in the lungs.
  (b) Is indicated in the treatment of lymphomas and testicular tumours.
  (c) Induced toxicity may necessitate administration of high concentrations of oxygen during anaesthesia.
  (d) Dosage has to be limited because of the risk of cardiomyopathy.
  (e) Administration may give rise to pyrexia.

225 (a) **False**   This is one of the fluoroquinolones that as a class have broad spectrum activity against Gram-negative organisms.
  (b) **True**   It has found a role in the treatment of infections in cystic fibrosis.
  (c) **False**   It raises theophylline concentrations increasing the possibility of theophylline toxicity.
  (d) **True**   For fear of damage to articular cartilages.
  (e) **False**

226 (a) **True**
  (b) **False**   In spite of its toxicity this is often the only life-saving agent for this condition, which is often found in the immunosuppressed patient.
  (c) **True**   It may also be useful in influenza.
  (d) **True**
  (e) **False**   This is the primary anti-viral agent used in the treatment of acquired immune deficiency syndrome (AIDS).

227 (a) **False**   Ziduvidine is converted to its triphosphate metabolite which then acts as a reverse transcriptase inhibitor.
  (b) **False**   It has to be administered every 4 hours because of its short half-life.
  (c) **True**
  (d) **False**   Neutropenia may be induced.
  (e) **True**   An increased incidence of blood abnormalities has been described.

228 (a) **False**   The indications for acyclovir are growing and it may be used on a long-term basis in the immunocompromised patient.
  (b) **True**
  (c) **False**   This is possibly a feature of ganciclovir.
  (d) **True**   Inosine pranobex has no direct antiviral action but stimulates the immune system.
  (e) **False**   Acyclovir and interferon alpha-2a are frequently used together in the treatment of Kaposi's sarcoma.

229 (a) **False**   Bleomycin is metabolized by a hydrolase that is not present in lung tissue (or skin); as a result lung (and skin) are major sites for toxicity.
  (b) **True**
  (c) **False**   The pulmonary toxicity is exacerbated by administration of high concentrations of oxygen. Even the normal inspired concentrations used during anaesthesia can result in a state of oxygen sensitivity; hence it is unwise to use elevated inspired oxygen concentrations in these patients.
  (d) **False**   The toxicity is mainly to the lungs.
  (e) **True**

230 Methotrexate:
   (a) Is absorbed from the gastrointestinal tract by an active transport system.
   (b) Is excreted primarily unchanged in the bile.
   (c) Should be administered simultaneously with leucovorin for maximum benefit.
   (d) Treatment contraindicates consumption of alcohol.
   (e) Dosage should be reduced in the presence of phenytoin.

231 Amphotericin:
   (a) Is mainly indicated in aspergillosis.
   (b) Is of no therapeutic value in infections due to *Histoplasma capsulatum*.
   (c) Is rarely associated with nephrotoxicity.
   (d) Is poorly absorbed from the gastrointestinal tract.
   (e) Is commonly associated with fever.

232 Fluconazole:
   (a) Is effective in the treatment of candidiasis.
   (b) Is effective in cryptococcal meningitis.
   (c) Acts by inhibiting energy production in the target organism.
   (d) May potentiate the effect of coumarin type anticoagulants.
   (e) Therapy may antagonize the effects of some oral hypoglycaemic agents.

233 Ketoconazole:
   (a) Unlike tioconazole, has no effect on human steroid synthesis.
   (b) Unlike fluconazole, may produce hepatic necrosis.
   (c) Unlike itraconazole, has no anti-testosterone activity.
   (d) Unlike griseofulvin, does not have gastrointestinal side-effects.
   (e) Unlike amphotercin, is not nephrotoxic.

Drugs and the endocrine system

234 In the endocrine system:
   (a) Prolactin secretion is suppressed by bromocriptine.
   (b) Prolactin secretion is stimulated by dopamine.
   (c) Antidiuretic hormone secretion is stimulated by morphine.
   (d) Fludrocortisol is least likely to cause sodium retention.
   (e) Carbamazepine suppresses antidiuretic hormone secretion.

230 (a) **True**   The active transport system, however, can get saturating in limited absorption after doses greater than 25–30 mg/m².

(b) **False**   It is mainly excreted through the kidneys by tubular secretion; hence drugs that inhibit secretion such as probenecid can lead to elevated plasma levels of methotrexate.

(c) **False**   Leucovorin should be given not less than 24 hours after methotrexate.

(d) **True**   Because of the risk of increased hepatotoxicity.

(e) **True**   Because of the displacement of methotrexate from plasma proteins.

231 (a) **False**   It may be resistant to amphotericin. Amphotericin is a broad spectrum antifungal agent that acts by binding to ergosterol, a component of fungal cell membranes, leading to loss of membrane integrity.

(b) **False**   Histoplasmosis is one of the indications for its use.

(c) **False**

(d) **True**

(e) **True**

232 (a) **True**   Especially in the immunocompromised patient.

(b) **True**

(c) **False**   It is an azole antifungal agent which acts by inhibiting fungal cytochrome P-450 to prevent the production of ergosterol, which is vital for the production and integrity of fungal membranes.

(d) **True**

(e) **False**   The effects of agents such as sulphonylureas may be increased because of elevated plasma concentrations.

233 (a) **False**   Ketoconazole and not tioconazole has adverse effects on steroid synthesis.

(b) **True**   Asymptomatic hepatotoxicity, sometimes progressing to hepatic failure, is a feature of ketoconazole.

(c) **False**   Ketoconazole is associated with gynaecomastia whereas itraconazole is not.

(d) **False**   They both show gastrointestinal tract side-effects.

(e) **True**

---

234 (a) **True**   Hence useful in the treatment of galactorrhoea.

(b) **False**

(c) **True**

(d) **False**   It is a potent retainer of sodium.

(e) **False**   It causes water retention especially in elderly patients with cardiac disease.

235 Adrenocorticotrophic hormone:
   (a) Is a glycoprotein released from the posterior pituitary gland.
   (b) Has a maximum adrenocortical effect that is at least ten times the basal output of the adrenal glands.
   (c) Is more likely to be associated with acne than prednisolone
   (d) Is as likely as prednisolone to lead to atrophy of the adrenal glands.
   (e) Administration preserves the patients' adrenal response to stress.

236 Vasopressin:
   (a) Acts on the proximal convoluted tubule to increase sodium reabsorption.
   (b) Can be administered nasally, orally, intramuscularly, intravenously or sub-cutaneously.
   (c) Is a potent splanchnic vasodilator.
   (d) Is the drug of choice for cranial diabetes insipidus.
   (e) Is preferably administered as a 'snuff'.

237 Calcitonin:
   (a) Is a 32-amino acid peptide secreted by the posterior pituitary.
   (b) Must be administered parenterally.
   (c) Accelerates the uptake of calcium from the gut.
   (d) May be used to treat the pain of Paget's disease.
   (e) May have a beneficial effect in vitamin D intoxication.

238 Danazol:
   (a) Has no effect on the hypothalamic-pituitary axis.
   (b) Inhibits the binding of oestrogens to their target cells.
   (c) Shows a poor correlation between biological effect and plasma half-life.
   (d) May be of use in hereditary angioneurotic oedema.
   (e) May be of use in porphyria.

235 (a) **False**   A polypeptide with 39 amino acids of which the first 24 confer bio-logical activity whereas the remainder confer species specificity.

   (b) **False**   About four times.

   (c) **True**   Because it will also stimulate the release of androgens.

   (d) **False**   Clearly it would lead to hypertrophy.

   (e) **False**   It suppresses the release of corticotrophin-releasing factor result-ing in failure of the hypothalamo-pituitary-adrenal axis.

236 (a) **False**   It acts on the distal tubules and the collecting ducts and does not increase sodium reabsorption.

   (b) **False**   Not orally as it would undergo enzymatic destruction.

   (c) **False**   It is a vasoconstrictor and is used by infusion in bleeding varices. Other side-effects include colic and exacerbation of angina.

   (d) **False**   It is too short acting. Nasally administered desmopressin would be the drug of choice. This agent is also unlikely to cause coro-nary artery spasm.

   (e) **False**   There is an association between the 'snuff' and bronchospasm and pulmonary fibrosis.

237 (a) **False**   It is a 32-peptide amino acid but is secreted by the thyroid and parathyroid glands.

   (b) **False**   It can be conveniently given via the intranasal route (which is associated with a lower incidence of adverse effects such as nausea and flushing). This is probably because less drug is actually reaching the systemic circulation, however.

   (c) **False**   It decreases the intestinal uptake of calcium and in a small way accelerates the renal loss of calcium. It can be used as a treat-ment for the hypercalcaemia of malignancy, as well as Paget's disease.

   (d) **True**   It is useful for both pain and hypercalcaemia.

   (e) **True**   By decreasing the level of plasma calcium and phosphate.

238 (a) **False**   Its action involves suppressing pituitary gonadotrophin secre-tion. It is an anabolic steroid, a 17-alpha alkyl derivative of tes-tosterone, with some androgenic activity.

   (b) **True**   Although this is not its primary action. It may also have actions on T-cell function since it has been shown to be useful in the treatment of idiopathic thrombocytopenic purpura.

   (c) **True**

   (d) **True**   It increases the synthesis of complement-esterase inhibitor.

   (e) **False**   It is contraindicated in this condition as it may increase ALA synthetase activity.

239 Bromocriptine:
   (a) Is a dopamine antagonist.
   (b) May be associated with a diminution in the size of pituitary micro-adenomas.
   (c) Can induce paranoid delusions.
   (d) Is a second line treatment in acromegaly.
   (e) May exacerbate primary hypertension.

240 Chlorpropamide:
   (a) Is useful in the treatment of the diabetes of chronic pancreatitis.
   (b) Stimulates glucose uptake into cells.
   (c) Has a useful appetite suppressing effect.
   (d) Is unsuitable for diabetics with renal disease.
   (e) Is especially useful in patients with mild cardiac failure as it is related to the thiazide diuretics.

241 Tolbutamide:
   (a) Is contraindicated in the elderly because of its long duration of action.
   (b) Is especially contraindicated in renal impairment.
   (c) May cause facial flushing in up to 20 per cent of patients after drinking alcohol.
   (d) Will only produce hypoglycaemia in a diabetic patient.
   (e) Will be less effective in patients on thiazide drugs.

242 Metformin:
   (a) Does not require functioning pancreatic tissue for its action.
   (b) Is useful in the alcoholic diabetic.
   (c) Is useful in the obese diabetic.
   (d) Is a useful drug in diabetics with compromised renal function.
   (e) May result in malabsorption of vitamin B_{12}.

243 Human insulin:
   (a) Is less likely to produce hypoglycaemia.
   (b) Absorption is most rapid from the abdominal wall.
   (c) Is less soluble than porcine insulin.
   (d) Should initially be given in smaller doses than animal insulins.
   (e) Has a shorter duration of action than animal insulins.

239 (a) **False** It is a dopamine agonist. This property makes it useful in the treatment of Parkinson's disease as it is similar to levodopa in its efficacy but with a lower incidence of nausea.

(b) **True** For prolactinomas and usually in men.

(c) **True** As it is derived from the ergot alkaloids. It can be looked upon as a derivative of lysergic acid diethylamide (LSD). Patients with Parkinson's disease may show such symptoms after treatment with this agent.

(d) **True** It can result in a paradoxical lowering of growth hormone concentrations, but is mainly used in patients unsuitable for surgery.

(e) **False** Its administration can initially be associated with postural hypotension.

240 (a) **False** The sulphonylurea drugs need functioning pancreatic tissue and act by increasing the response of islet cells to glucose.

(b) **True** In cells in the muscle.

(c) **False** It stimulates appetite.

(d) **True** Among the sulphonylurea compounds chlorpropamide is notable because it is excreted unchanged by the kidneys.

(e) **False** It is indeed related to the thiazides but by potentiating the effects of antidiuretic hormone it leads to dilutional hyponatraemia.

241 (a) **False** It is useful in the elderly because of its short half-life.

(b) **False** It is a useful anti-diabetic in patients with renal disease as it is principally metabolized in the liver.

(c) **False** It is chlorpropamide that is typically associated with facial flushing after consuming alcohol. However, alcohol may increase the hypoglycaemic effect of tolbutamide and in a few patients may show an antabuse-like effect.

(d) **False**

(e) **True** Thiazide drugs tend to antagonize the effects of tolbutamide.

242 (a) **True** It is effective even without a functioning pancreas. It tends not to cause hypoglycaemia in non-diabetics.

(b) **False** Because of the increased risk of lactic acidosis.

(c) **True** As it tends to produce anorexia. It may however also reduce vitamin B_{12} absorption.

(d) **False** Due to the risk of lactic acidosis.

(e) **True**

243 (a) **False** It produces hypoglycaemia with the same or even greater frequency as other types of insulin because of poor penetration across the blood–brain barrier, and a lower catecholamine release in response to hypoglycaemia.

(b) **True**

(c) **False** It is more soluble and less antigenic.

(d) **True** Because of the greater possibility of hypoglycaemia with it.

(e) **True**

244 Carbimazole:
   (a) Is a prodrug.
   (b) Suppresses thyroxine secretion.
   (c) Takes more than 2–3 weeks for exerting its effect.
   (d) Is associated with leucopenia in 3–5 per cent of treated patients.
   (e) Is absolutely contraindicated in pregnancy.

245 Prostaglandins:
   (a) Are 20-carbon unsaturated fatty acids.
   (b) Are stored in the prostate gland.
   (c) Of class $PGF_{2\alpha}$ cause uterine relaxation.
   (d) Of class E_2 cause uterine contraction.
   (e) Of class PGI_2 cause vasodilatation.

246 Comparing the use of oxytocin and ergometrine in labour:
   (a) Oxytocin is associated with a transient decrease in systolic blood pressure
        while ergometrine may give rise to a marked increase in it.
   (b) Ergometrine is associated with a sustained increase in central venous
        pressure whereas oxytocin causes a reduction in it.
   (c) They are equally effective at reducing blood loss at delivery.
   (d) Both are associated with nausea.
   (e) Both are used for the induction of labour.

247 Ethinyloestradiol:
   (a) May prevent osteoporosis.
   (b) Is a useful treatment for endometrial hyperplasia.
   (c) Is associated with decreased blood antithrombin III levels.
   (d) Unlike the progesterone-only preparations, is suitable for use in patients
        with hypertension.
   (e) Is associated with the same risk of thromboembolism as the progesterone-
        only preparations.

244 (a) **True** It is hydrolysed to methimazole for its effect.
   (b) **False** It leads to blockage of iodination of tyrosol residues and prevents thyroid hormone production.
   (c) **True** It does not prevent secretion but interferes with the production of thyroid hormones.
   (d) **False** It occurs very infrequently (approximately one in 500 patients).
   (e) **False** Antithyroid drugs can be given if surgery is not undertaken. The baby may, however, be born with a goitre.

245 (a) **True** They are called 'eicosanoids' because they are derivatives of polyunsaturated eicosanoic (C_{20}) fatty acids and are powerful local tissue hormones.
   (b) **False** There is no storage site for these compounds. They are produced as required, by the action of phospholipase A_2 on cell membrane. Arachidonic acid is liberated and is used as a substrate for lipooxygenase to yield the precursors of the leukotrienes or by cyclo-oxygenase to yield the precursors of prostaglandins.
   (c) **False** These are present in menstrual fluid and may actually cause dysmenorrhoea.
   (d) **True** These may be used to induce abortion.
   (e) **True** This group is represented by prostacyclin, one of the most effective inhibitors of platelet aggregation available, in addition to being a powerful vasodilator.

246 (a) **True**
   (b) **False** Both produce an increase in CVP, more so with ergometrine.
   (c) **True** Although they differ in the time course of their effects.
   (d) **False** It is a feature of ergometrine.
   (e) **False** Ergometrine is not used for this purpose as it can produce prolonged tonic contractions of the uterus causing a severe reduction in placental blood flow.

247 (a) **True** Making it useful in hormone replacement therapy.
   (b) **False** It is contraindicated in this condition.
   (c) **True** Increasing the risk of deep venous thrombosis.
   (d) **False**
   (e) **False** Progesterone-only preparations have a lower risk of thromboembolism and may be used as an alternative form of contraception in patients coming for surgery.

248 Disodium etidronate:
   (a) Should be given with milk to avoid dyspepsia.
   (b) May induce hyperphosphataemia.
   (c) Reduces serum alfacalcidol levels to normal in Paget's disease.
   (d) Inhibits osteoclastic bone resorption.
   (e) May cause defective bone mineralization.

249 Calcitriol:
   (a) Is contraindicated in anephric patients.
   (b) May cause nausea and vomiting in overdose.
   (c) Is an effective treatment in pseudohypoparathyroidism.
   (d) Is as effective an antirachitic agent as alfacalcidol.
   (e) Should be administered with calcium for best effect.

250 In the management of osteoporosis it is claimed that:
   (a) Hormone replacement therapy with progesterone is an effective preventative treatment.
   (b) Sodium fluoride may be helpful.
   (c) 1,25-dihydroxycholecalciferol (calcitriol) is of proven benefit.
   (d) Calcitonin treatment accelerates bone loss.
   (e) Etidronate may be of some benefit.

251 Oestradiol administered in the postmenopausal period:
   (a) Simulates physiological activity better as a transdermal preparation than when administered orally.
   (b) Is not associated with an increased risk of myocardial infarction.
   (c) Must be administered with progesterone to reduce the incidence of stroke.
   (d) Has no effect on the incidence of endometrial neoplasia.
   (e) As a transdermal preparation results in elevated levels of clotting factors.

248 (a) **False** Because the absorption of an already poorly absorbed drug is further reduced. Moreover it does not usually cause dyspepsia.

(b) **True** Not common, however.

(c) **False** Serum alfacalcidol levels are not raised in Paget's disease and are not altered by etidronate.

(d) **True** Etidronate is one of the bisphosphonates which are analogues of pyrophosphate binding strongly to hydroxyapatite crystals to inhibit bone mineral dissolution. They will also, however, inhibit bone mineralization. Other members of the group are clodronic acid and pamidronic acid, both more potent than etidronate.

(e) **True** See above.

249 (a) **False** Vitamin D precursors in the diet or from the effects of ultraviolet light on the skin undergo hydroxylation in the liver to produce 25-hydroxycholecalciferol. Parathormone acts on renal 1-alpha-hydroxylase to encourage the production of 1,25-dihydroxycholecalciferol (calcitriol) the active agent in preventing rickets. Calcitriol administered orally does not depend on renal metabolism and so is useful in the anephric.

(b) **True** Because of its ability to induce the adverse effects of hypercalcaemia.

(c) **True**

(d) **True** Calcitriol has a short half-life however, therefore if administration is irregular plasma calcium concentrations will fluctuate. Hence alfacalcidol (which undergoes hydroxylation to calcitriol in the liver) or even calciferol are used more often.

(e) **False** Because of the risk of hypercalcaemia.

250 (a) **False** It is oestrogens that have a beneficial effect.

(b) **True** But may lead to mineralization defects.

(c) **False** This is of doubtful value and maybe risky.

(d) **False** This hormone will inhibit bone resorption but must be administered parenterally.

(e) **True** The biphosphonates are potent inhibitors of bone resorption and in the short term have been shown to decrease the incidence of refracture in patients with spinal osteoporosis.

251 (a) **True** Because of the hepatic first-pass effect after oral administration.

(b) **True**

(c) **False**

(d) **False** This is why progesterone is added in hormone replacement therapy.

(e) **False** This happens with the use of oral preparations due to the effect on hepatic metabolism increasing the clotting factors.

252 Demeclocycline:
    (a) Is effective in the treatment of acne.
    (b) Has anti-anabolic effects.
    (c) Administration increases the requirement of coumarin-type anticoagulants.
    (d) Treatment may result in raised intracranial pressure.
    (e) Treatment may lead to chronic hyponatraemia.

253 Tamoxifen:
    (a) Is an oestrogen agonist.
    (b) Is particularly effective against liver secondaries in breast neoplasia.
    (c) May exacerbate the pain of bony metastases.
    (d) Can induce thrombocytaemia.
    (e) Increases the requirement of coumarin-type anticoagulants when the two are administered at the same time.

254 Goserelin:
    (a) Results in an acute decrease in serum testosterone levels.
    (b) Reduces bone pain shortly after administration.
    (c) Should not be co-administered with cyproterone.
    (d) Is not as effective as orchidectomy in tumour suppression.
    (e) Therapy is complicated by an increased risk of deep venous thrombosis.

255 Cyproterone:
    (a) Inhibits spermatogenesis.
    (b) Causes the regression of gynaecomastia.
    (c) May lead to aberrant sexual behaviour
    (d) Is the anti-androgen agent of choice in adolescents.
    (e) Leads to sedation.

256 Prolonged hydrocortisone therapy:
    (a) May lead to osteomalacia.
    (b) May lead to growth retardation in children.
    (c) May lead to euphoria.
    (d) May lead to polycythaemia.
    (e) May lead to muscle fasciculations and even contractures.

252 (a) **True** As it belongs to the group of tetracyclines.
(b) **True** It will tend to raise blood urea levels especially in those with renal impairment.
(c) **False** The tetracyclines depress plasma prothrombin activity and so reduced doses of anticoagulants may be required.
(d) **True** This is one of the types of drugs that can cause benign intracranial hypertension.
(e) **False** It may be beneficial particularly if hyponatraemia is due to inappropriate antidiuretic hormone secretion.

253 (a) **False** It is a non-steroidal anti-oestrogen agent which binds to cytoplasmic oestrogen receptors to form a complex that blocks the access of oestrogen to the receptors.
(b) **False** Not usually against secondaries in the liver.
(c) **True**
(d) **False** Thrombocytopenia has been reported, although it may resolve without the drug being stopped.
(e) **False** It potentiates the action of the anticoagulant.

254 (a) **False** It is a synthetic analogue of gonadotrophin releasing hormone. It stimulates the testosterone release initially but on chronic administration it mimics the effects of orchidectomy.
(b) **False** See (a) above. A temporary exacerbation in symptoms may be prevented by the use of an anti-androgen agent.
(c) **False** It can be administered with cyproterone to prevent the temporary exacerbation of symptoms due to goserelin administration.
(d) **False** Goserelin which incidently is given by depot injection produces comparable reduction in serum testosterone levels to orchidectomy. (Buserelin is an alternative to goserelin and can be given intranasally.
(e) **False** Unlike oestrogens.

255 (a) **True** This is reversible, however.
(b) **False** It may actually lead to gynaecomastia and rarely to galactorrhoea and benign breast nodules.
(c) **False** It may actually control it.
(d) **False** It should be avoided in this age group as it may arrest bone maturation and testicular development.
(e) **True** And may produce impaired ability to drive and operate machines.

256 (a) **False** It is osteoporosis.
(b) **True** This may be due to inhibitory effects on DNA synthesis and cell division.
(c) **True** Or depression.
(d) **True** There is an increase in haemoglobin and red cell content.
(e) **False** A myopathy with weakness of the proximal muscles of arms and legs may occur.

257 Prednisolone:
   (a) Suppresses antibody production.
   (b) Decreases the number of circulating lymphocytes.
   (c) Has no effect on the late manifestations of inflammation.
   (d) Shows enhanced activity in renal failure.
   (e) Shows reduced activity in mild liver disease.

258 Compared to hydrocortisone:
   (a) Prednisolone has twice the anti-inflammatory activity.
   (b) Prednisolone has one-tenth the mineralocorticoid activity.
   (c) Betamethasone has 25 times the anti-inflammatory activity.
   (d) The mineralocorticoid activity of dexamethasone is about 25 per cent.
   (e) Fludrocortisone has about ten times the anti-inflammatory activity.

Drugs and the blood

259 Heparin:
   (a) Has no effect on the intrinsic coagulation system.
   (b) Is destroyed in interacting with thrombin.
   (c) Shows increased dose requirements in pulmonary embolism in comparison with normal individuals.
   (d) Is required in only small doses to prevent thrombin formation.
   (e) Catalyses the effects of antithrombin III on thrombin and factor XII_a.

260 Heparin:
   (a) Is a gluconated basic mucopolysaccharide.
   (b) Is eliminated from the body according to first order kinetics.
   (c) Can result in toxicity to the baby during breast feeding.
   (d) Does not cross the placenta.
   (e) Excretion is markedly increased in hypothermia.

261 Heparin therapy:
   (a) Can be complicated by thrombocytopenia.
   (b) May be useful in the therapy of hyperlipidaemia.
   (c) Can be complicated by hirsutism.
   (d) Of very long duration can lead to osteomalacia.
   (e) May be complicated by hypoaldosteronism.

257 (a) **False** It acts as an immunosuppressant by suppressing the thymus-dependent T lymphocytes and not antibody production.
   (b) **True** Particular activity is against helper cells.
   (c) **False** Just like cortisol it inhibits the late manifestations such as deposition of collagen, proliferation of fibroblasts and cicatrization.
   (d) **True** Because of the reduced levels of transcortin and albumin.
   (e) **False** The half-life is prolonged due to lower levels of binding proteins.

258 (a) **False** It is four times.
   (b) **False** It is approximately 80 per cent of the activity of hydrocortisone.
   (c) **True**
   (d) **False** Dexamethasone has very little mineralocorticoid effect.
   (e) **True** Although its mineralocorticoid activity is more than 100 times that of hydrocortisone.

---

259 (a) **False** Heparin prolongs the whole blood clotting time. It accelerates the interaction between antithrombin III and several proteases in the coagulation cascade, including factor X_a without which neither intrinsic nor extrinsic coagulation pathways can function.
   (b) **False**
   (c) **True** They show increased heparin clearance.
   (d) **True** As a result low doses of heparin have a prophylactic role in the prevention of thromboembolism. Larger doses are required to actually inhibit thrombin once it is formed.
   (e) **True**

260 (a) **False** It is an acidic sulphated mucopolysaccharide.
   (b) **True** However the half-life is dose-dependent varying from 1 hour with a 100 units/kg dose to 5 hours with a 800 units/kg dose.
   (c) **False** Heparin is neither excreted in breast milk nor absorbed after oral administration.
   (d) **True** It is a relatively big, highly polar molecule with a molecular weight of 6,000–20,000.
   (e) **False**

261 (a) **True** In about 10 per cent of patients after 5 days or more of therapy. The mechanism of this effect is unclear but may involve heparin-dependent antiplatelet antibodies.
   (b) **True** By releasing lipoprotein lipase into the circulation. However, rebound hyperlipaemia may occur when the therapy is stopped.
   (c) **False** In fact alopecia can occur.
   (d) **False** It may result in osteoporosis.
   (e) **True**

262 Protamine:
  (a) Is administered in a dose of 10 mg to counteract the effects of every 1000 units of heparin.
  (b) May lead to adverse effects in insulin-dependent diabetics treated with certain long-acting insulin preparations.
  (c) Is not known to give rise to pulmonary hypertension in man.
  (d) Rarely causes marked hypotension even when injected rapidly.
  (e) Should be given by rapid bolus injection as it is avidly protein bound.

263 Enoxaparin:
  (a) Has thrombin inhibitory activity equivalent to standard preparations of heparin.
  (b) Remains active against factor X_a even at low concentrations.
  (c) Has better subcutaneous absorption than unfractionated heparin.
  (d) Is more likely than unfractionated heparin to result in bleeding complications.
  (e) Has no effect on lipoprotein lipase.

264 Warfarin:
  (a) Acts by preventing the synthesis of factors II, IV and XI by preventing gammacarboxylation of glutamic acid.
  (b) Is 60 per cent protein bound.
  (c) Is an abortifacient.
  (d) May produce skin necrosis in vitamin C deficiency.
  (e) Produces clinically beneficial anticoagulant effect within 5–6 hours of oral administration.

265 Ancrod:
  (a) Is a pro-coagulant accelerating the conversion of fibrinogen into fibrin.
  (b) Is useful in antagonizing the effects of heparin in individuals sensitive to protamine.
  (c) Reduces blood viscosity.
  (d) May be used in the prevention of recurrent subarachnoid haemorrhage.
  (e) Has a very long duration of action.

262 (a) **True**   Particularly if the action of heparin is to be reversed within 3–4 hours of its administration. A lower dose of protamine may be given after several hours of heparin administration unless there is evidence of impaired clotting.

     (b) **True**   Because of sensitization, if a protamine containing insulin preparation had been used previously.

     (c) **False**   Increased concentrations of thromboxane A_2 and its metabolites, which may result from protamine administration, cause intense pulmonary vasoconstriction and pulmonary hypertension.

     (d) **False**   It can cause hypotension because of the same reasons as in (c) above and also histamine liberation.

     (e) **False**   It should be administered slowly preferably at no more than 20 mg/minute.

263 (a) **False**   Enoxaparin is a heparin fragment with a molecular weight of 5500 or less. It has much less antithrombin activity but much the same ability to potentiate the inhibition of factor X_a. This may be one of the reasons why there is less tendency to bleed with it and yet it retains good prophylactic activity against hypercoagulability. It is also less likely to exhibit the antiplatelet activity of unfractionated heparin.

     (b) **True**   It may release endogenous heparin.

     (c) **True**   Because of a low molecular weight.

     (d) **False**   (See (a) above.)

     (e) **False**   It is the same as with unfractionated heparin.

264 (a) **False**   It is the prevention of carboxylation of factors II, VII, IX and X.

     (b) **False**   It is 97 per cent. This has implications for drug interactions.

     (c) **True**   Particularly in early pregnancy.

     (d) **True**   Especially if large doses are used.

     (e) **False**   Warfarin acts by inhibiting the production of factors II, VII, IX and X; the half-lives of these factors range from 6–60 hours, hence it would normally take some days for clinical effect. The greatest effect is related to the activity of factor X which has a half-life of 40 hours.

265 (a) **False**   It is an anticoagulant derived from Malayan pit viper venom. Although it accelerates the conversion of fibrinogen to fibrin, this fibrin is quite unstable thus causing anticoagulation.

     (b) **False**   It is an alternative to heparin.

     (c) **True**

     (d) **False**   It increases the risk of bleeding.

     (e) **True**   But there is a relatively lower risk of bleeding.

266 Streptokinase:
   (a) Is a direct plasminogen activator.
   (b) Resistance may develop during therapy.
   (c) Acts only at the site of an existing clot.
   (d) Therapy may be complicated by pyrexia.
   (e) Is useful for the lysis of intraocular clots.

267 Tissue-type plasminogen activator (alteplase):
   (a) Gives rise to indiscriminate plasminogen activation.
   (b) Produces less fibrinolysis than streptokinase.
   (c) Is non-antigenic.
   (d) Has a longer duration of action than streptokinase.
   (e) Is prone to cause severe systemic hypotensive reactions.

268 Tranexamic acid:
   (a) Is more potent than epsilon aminocaproic acid.
   (b) Can only be used intravenously.
   (c) May lead to failure of recanalization of venous thrombi.
   (d) May be of value in haemophilia.
   (e) Reduces the incidence of rebleeding in subarachnoid haemorrhage.

269 An appropriate use:
   (a) Of factor VII is for von Willebrand's disease.
   (b) Of factor IX is for haemophilia B.
   (c) Of fresh frozen plasma is for congenital deficiency of factor V.
   (d) Of cryoprecipitate is for microvascular bleeding with a fibrinogen level below 0.5 g/litre.
   (e) Of fresh frozen plasma is in microvascular bleeding with a fibrinogen level over 0.8 g/litre.

270 Antiplatelet agent:
   (a) Dipyridamole acts as an irreversible cyclo-oxygenase inhibitor.
   (b) Dipyridamole should not be administered simultaneously with warfarin.
   (c) Sulphinpyrazone acts by blocking the synthesis of prostaglandins and allied substances.
   (d) Aspirin is an irreversible phosphodiesterase inhibitor.
   (e) Prostacyclin acts via stimulation of platelet adenyl cyclase.

266 (a) **False** It acts indirectly by combining with plasminogen creating an activator complex resulting in the conversion of plasminogen to plasmin. Plasmin is a protease enzyme which accelerates fibrin degradation. It is urokinase, which is a direct plasminogen activator.

(b) **True** Because of formation of streptokinase antibodies.

(c) **False** There is systemic fibrinolysis.

(d) **True**

(e) **False** A less antigenic agent is indicated. Urokinase has been considered the more suitable alternative.

267 (a) **False** This agent has a high affinity for fibrin and produces a relative clot-selective activation of plasminogen.

(b) **True** In equipotent doses.

(c) **True** As it is a natural product made by recombinant DNA technology.

(d) **False** Its duration of action is shorter. This may result in a higher incidence of rethrombosis.

(e) **False** These are more a feature of streptokinase.

268 (a) **True** It is a more potent fibrinolytic inhibitor by a factor of 10. Plasminogen interacts with fibrin via lysine-binding sites that can be blocked competitively by antifibrinolytic agents to inhibit plasminogen activation.

(b) **False** It can be given orally if treatment lasts more than 3 days.

(c) **True** Clotting without fibrinolysis leads to fibrosis.

(d) **True** This is of prophylactic value in such patients when they are undergoing procedures such as dental extractions.

(e) **True** But it may not reduce death rates.

269 (a) **False** Factor VII is useful for the treatment of its congenital deficiency or overdose of oral anticoagulants.

(b) **True** This is prothrombin complex concentrate.

(c) **True** There are few absolute indications for using fresh frozen plasma despite its widespread use .

(d) **True** This contains factors VIII, XIII, fibronectin, fibrinogen, and von Willibrand's factor.

(e) **True** Microvascular bleeding is manifested as a continuing ooze from surgical wounds and puncture sites. If the patient has a prolonged prothrombin time but an adequate fibrinogen level the bleeding may be due to a relative lack of factors VIII and V, which can be provided by fresh frozen plasma.

270 (a) **False** It is a phosphodiesterase inhibitor which prevents platelet aggregation by increasing cyclic-AMP levels.

(b) **False** This is a useful combination used frequently in patients with prosthetic heart valves.

(c) **True**

(d) **False** It is an irreversible cyclo-oxygenase inhibitor.

(e) **True**

271 Compound sodium lactate solution:
   (a) Contains 154 mmol/litre of sodium.
   (b) Is hypertonic in comparison to 0.9 per cent saline.
   (c) Has the same osmolarity as 5 per cent dextrose.
   (d) Has the same pH as 5 per cent dextrose.
   (e) Only contains sodium, potassium and calcium cations.

272 8.4 per cent sodium bicarbonate:
   (a) Should be administered routinely from early on during cardiopulmonary resuscitation.
   (b) May cause paradoxical acidosis.
   (c) Increases tissue oxygen delivery.
   (d) Is useful in the hyponatraemia of the 'sick cell' syndrome.
   (e) Can be administered subcutaneously if venous access is impossible.

273 In colloids:
   (a) The weight average molecular weight (Mw) of gelatins is greater than their number average molecular weight (Mn).
   (b) The weight average molecular weight is more directly related to the oncotic activity than the number average molecular weight.
   (c) The number average and weight average molecular weights are identical for succinylated gelatin but not urea-linked gelatin.
   (d) Polydispersity has no advantage.
   (e) Such as albumin solution, the clinician has a naturally-derived polydisperse colloid.

274 Among the commonly used colloids:
   (a) Apart from dilutional effects, only dextran shows anti-coagulant properties.
   (b) Urea-linked gelatin has one of the lowest incidence of allergic reactions.
   (c) Hydroxyethyl starch has one of the lowest incidence of allergic reactions.
   (d) Only dextran 70 should not be mixed with citrated blood.
   (e) Succinylated gelatin has a longer half-life in the circulation than urea-linked gelatin.

271 (a) **False** It contains approximately 131 mmol/litre of sodium.
   (b) **False** Its tonicity is marginally lower.
   (c) **True** The difference is negligible (280 versus 278 mosmol/litre).
   (d) **False** 5 per cent dextrose is much more acidic and this may be important when drugs are added to 5 per cent dextrose.
   (e) **True**

272 (a) **False** The guidelines for the use of sodium bicarbonate have been revised because, during efficient cardiopulmonary resuscitation, significant acidaemia is slow to occur.
   (b) **True** Although the clinical significance of this is open to debate. It may be due to the passage of carbon dioxide, which is liberated from sodium bicarbonate, across the blood–brain barrier or into the cells to induce acidosis.
   (c) **False** The oxygen dissociation curve is shifted to the left resulting in decreased oxygen delivery.
   (d) **False** Administration of sodium in this case is dangerous because of increased sodium load.
   (e) **False** It is very irritant and may cause tissue necrosis.

273 (a) **True** Because gelatins usually contain a range of molecules of differing molecular weights. The average molecular weight of such 'polydisperse colloids' may be classified according to the weight average or the number average. Weight average molecular weight will always be greater since the larger molecules contribute more to the measured effect than the smaller ones.
   (b) **False** Number average values are more directly related to oncotic activity.
   (c) **False** These are polydisperse colloids each containing molecules with a range of weights.
   (d) **False** It is possible that smaller molecules produce initial plasma expansion, decrease viscosity and then promote a diuresis. Larger molecules sustain the effect.
   (e) **False** In albumin solutions the molecules are of equal size; the number average and weight average molecular weights are hence the same.

274 (a) **False** Hydroxyethyl starch, if given in volumes greater than 1 litre, reduces the levels of factor VIII. Additionally it has an appreciable fibrinolytic effect.
   (b) **False** It has one of the highest incidences.
   (c) **True**
   (d) **False** Urea-linked gelatin contains calcium, will clot citrated blood and under the right circumstances will also gel fresh frozen plasma.
   (e) **False** Both have a half-life of about 2.5 hours.

275 Pentastarch:
   (a) Is prepared as a 10 per cent solution in 5 per cent dextrose.
   (b) Has a plasma half-life of 1.5–2 hours as in the case of hetastarch.
   (c) Will interfere with cross-matching determinations when used in amounts greater than 10 per cent of blood volume .
   (d) May prolong the prothrombin time.
   (e) Is minimally excreted through the kidney.

276 Oxpentifylline:
   (a) Has weak alpha adrenoreceptor blocking properties.
   (b) Inhibits red cell deformation.
   (c) Unlike naftidrofuryl enhances cellular metabolism in ischaemic tissues.
   (d) May intensify the hypoglycaemic action of insulin.
   (e) May have a role in the management of endotoxaemia.

277 Iron:
   (a) In haemoglobin constitutes 20 per cent of total body iron stores.
   (b) Absorption from the gut is better using the ferric formulation.
   (c) Absorption is independent of the source of the iron.
   (d) Uptake occurs in the stomach, hence the anaemia of partial gastrectomy.
   (e) Excretion is principally via the kidney.

278 Iron:
   (a) As ferrous gluconate is the preparation with the least side-effects.
   (b) Replacement in iron deficiency anaemia results in an increase in the haemoglobin concentration of 0.1 g/dl/day.
   (c) If given parenterally results in a faster response in anaemia.
   (d) Is the treatment of choice for all hypochromic anaemias.
   (e) As iron sorbitol citric acid is the preferred intravenous formulation of iron.

279 Vitamin B_{12}:
   (a) Is abundant in leafy vegetables.
   (b) Requirements in humans are supplied to an extent of 10 per cent by colonic bacteria.
   (c) Is stored complexed to transcobalamin I.
   (d) Undergoes enterohepatic recirculation resulting in decreased total absorption.
   (e) Daily requirements are 3–5 μg.

275 (a) **False** It is prepared in 0.9 per cent saline.
   (b) **False** Both have relatively long half-lives, in the region of 20 hours.
   (c) **False** It can, however, result in rouleaux formation.
   (d) **True** As will many other plasma expanders.
   (e) **False** Kidney is the main route of excretion.

276 (a) **True** This makes it additionally useful in patients with peripheral vascular disease.
   (b) **False** It is supposed to enhance red cell deformation.
   (c) **False** Naftidrofuryl (Praxilene) is claimed to aid energy production in hypoxic conditions.
   (d) **True** Not only for insulin but also oral hypoglycaemic agents. It is an uncommon occurrence but may be important because the drug is intended for use in patients with peripheral vascular disease who often also have diabetes.
   (e) **True** The drug may have a role in preventing the generation of tumour necrosis factor.

277 (a) **False** 70 per cent of total body iron is in haemoglobin.
   (b) **False** Inorganic ferrous iron is better absorbed.
   (c) **False** Iron provided by the animal sources is better absorbed than iron presented in cereal crops.
   (d) **False** Gastric acid enhances iron absorption, which actually takes place in the small intestine.
   (e) **False** Absorbed iron is rarely excreted.

278 (a) **False** Side-effects are not dependent on the preparation but on the dose of elemental iron.
   (b) **False** It usually takes about 5 days before reticulocyte response and increase in haemoglobin are observed.
   (c) **False** The response time is the same, parenteral administration only circumvents poor compliance or malabsorption.
   (d) **False**
   (e) **False** This is an intramuscular preparation.

279 (a) **False** Liver and heart are the main sources.
   (b) **False** Although colonic bacteria make vitamin B_{12}, the site of formation is too far from the site of absorption.
   (c) **True**
   (d) **False** Enterohepatic re-circulation improves the uptake form the gut.
   (e) **True**

280 Vitamin B_{12}:
   (a) Given during continuous exposure to nitrous oxide reverses any tendency to leucopenia.
   (b) As hydroxocobalamin is the preferred replacement therapy in deficiency states.
   (c) Treatment may be associated with cardiac arrhythmias.
   (d) Is required in doses of greater than 2000 μg/day for the treatment of subacute combined degeneration of the cord.
   (e) Restores vision in tobacco amblyopia.

281 Folic acid:
   (a) Is only found in animal tissues.
   (b) Is stored in the liver, with a 4-month reserve.
   (c) Will prevent neurological changes of subacute combined degeneration.
   (d) Antagonizes the toxic effects of sulphonamides in humans.
   (e) Is used in 'folic acid rescue' from high-dose methotrexate therapy.

282 Magnesium sulphate:
   (a) Can produce cardiac arrest in diastole.
   (b) Is a useful tocolytic agent.
   (c) Is a directly acting vasoconstrictor.
   (d) Has a curare-like effect.
   (e) Is considered contraindicated in patients with myocardial infarction.

283 In Raynaud's syndrome:
   (a) Nifedipine reduces the frequency of attacks.
   (b) Thymoxamine is of no benefit.
   (c) Captopril is of benefit in patients with primary Raynaud's disease.
   (d) Ketanserin may be of value.
   (e) Eicosapentaenoic acid is the treatment of first choice.

284 Hyperlipidaemia can result from intake of:
   (a) Labetalol.
   (b) Captopril.
   (c) Chlorthalidone.
   (d) Combination of propranolol and hydrochlorthiazide.
   (e) Probucol.

280 (a) **False**   Treatment with vitamin B_{12} has no effect. B_{12} is a co-factor in the action of methionine synthase, which is involved in the nitrous oxide-vitamin interaction. A by-product of the activity of this enzyme is tetrahydrofolate, which is involved in the production of deoxythymidine, a vital constituent of DNA. It is by providing an alternate source of tetrahydrofolate such as folinic acid (5-formyl tetrahydrofolate) that will prevent megaloblastic changes and leucopenia in patients exposed to nitrous oxide.

  (b) **True**   This is retained longer in the body than cyanocobalamin.

  (c) **True**   In patients with hypokalaemia.

  (d) **False**   Such large doses are not required.

  (e) **False**   Only the blood picture is restored.

281 (a) **False**   Also found in leafy vegetables.

  (b) **True**

  (c) **False**   It will make these worse.

  (d) **False**   Sulphonamides prevent the bacterial manufacture of folic acid, however toxic effects of sulphonamides in humans are not related to metabolism of folic acid. Moreover humans usually take folic acid as a vitamin in their diet.

  (e) **False**   Methotrexate inhibits dihydrofolate reductase preventing tetrahydrofolate production, which must be provided in the form of folinic acid to prevent toxicity.

282 (a) **True**

  (b) **True**   Although not in current UK practice.

  (c) **False**   It is a directly acting vasodilator.

  (d) **True**   Possibly interacting with the non-depolarizing neuromuscular blocking agents.

  (e) **False**   Combination of magnesium sulphate, nitrates and ACE inhibitors may reduce mortality after myocardial infarction.

283 (a) **True**

  (b) **False**   Its alpha-adrenergic blocking properties are useful in this condition.

  (c) **True**   Because of vasodilatatory actions.

  (d) **True**   It is a vasodilator.

  (e) **False**   It is useful for the reduction of plasma triglycerides.

284 (a) **False**   This combined alpha- and beta-adrenoceptor blocking agent has little effect on lipids.

  (b) **False**   Absence of causing hyperlipidaemia is considered an advantage.

  (c) **True**   Especially when given to younger patients who may be much more likely to develop an unfavourable lipid profile.

  (d) **True**   A combination that is prone to produce an elevation in triglycerides.

  (e) **False**   This increases the faecal excretion of bile acids and produces about a 10 per cent decrease in low-density lipoprotein levels, but with no effect on triglycerides. However prolongation of the QT interval is a possible disadvantage.

285 In the drug treatment of hyperlipidaemia:
  (a) Acipimox is appropriate for type IIa hyperlipidaemia.
  (b) Cholestyramine is appropriate for type IV hyperlipidaemia.
  (c) Fenofibrate is appropriate for type III hyperlipidaemia.
  (d) Colestipol is appropriate for type II hyperlipidaemia.
  (e) Nicotinic acid is of no value in type V hyperlipidaemia.

286 Among the lipid-lowering agents:
  (a) Pravastatin acts as a hydroxyl-methyl-glutaryl coenzyme A reductase inhibitor.
  (b) Bezafibrate suppresses endogenous cholesterol synthesis.
  (c) Nicofuranose acts as an anion exchange resin.
  (d) Gemfibrozil acts by activating lipoprotein lipase.
  (e) Simvastatin acts as an anion exchange resin.

General pharmacology and statistics

287 Absorption:
  (a) By facilitated diffusion is independent of the concentration gradient.
  (b) Of salicylates from the gastrointestinal tract is mainly by passive diffusion.
  (c) By diffusion is limited by the capacity of the capillary wall for diffusion rather than the tissue blood flow.
  (d) By passive diffusion is selective for lipid-soluble compounds.
  (e) By passive diffusion is independent of the concentration gradient.

288 Bioavailability:
  (a) Is proportional to the first-pass effect.
  (b) Defines the amount of drug absorbed after oral administration.
  (c) Of orally administered propranolol is usually over 60 per cent.
  (d) Of intramuscularly administered phenytoin is more than 95 per cent.
  (e) Of digoxin is dependent on the formulation used.

289 The volume of distribution:
  (a) Of a drug is independent of changes in cardiac output.
  (b) Of heparin is approximately 40 litres in a 70 kg man.
  (c) Cannot be greater than total body water.
  (d) Is dependent on the degree of protein binding.
  (e) In first order kinetics is equivalent to the dose of the drug divided by the product of the elimination rate constant and area under the plasma concentration time curve.

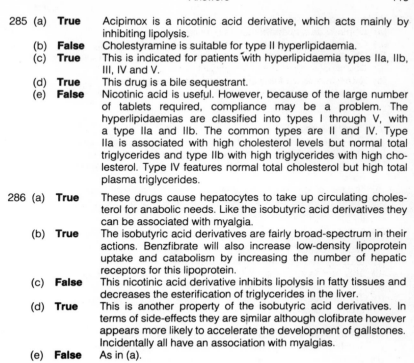

285 (a) **True**   Acipimox is a nicotinic acid derivative, which acts mainly by inhibiting lipolysis.

(b) **False**   Cholestyramine is suitable for type II hyperlipidaemia.

(c) **True**   This is indicated for patients with hyperlipidaemia types IIa, IIb, III, IV and V.

(d) **True**   This drug is a bile sequestrant.

(e) **False**   Nicotinic acid is useful. However, because of the large number of tablets required, compliance may be a problem. The hyperlipidaemias are classified into types I through V, with a type IIa and IIb. The common types are II and IV. Type IIa is associated with high cholesterol levels but normal total triglycerides and type IIb with high triglycerides with high cholesterol. Type IV features normal total cholesterol but high total plasma triglycerides.

286 (a) **True**   These drugs cause hepatocytes to take up circulating cholesterol for anabolic needs. Like the isobutyric acid derivatives they can be associated with myalgia.

(b) **True**   The isobutyric acid derivatives are fairly broad-spectrum in their actions. Benzfibrate will also increase low-density lipoprotein uptake and catabolism by increasing the number of hepatic receptors for this lipoprotein.

(c) **False**   This nicotinic acid derivative inhibits lipolysis in fatty tissues and decreases the esterification of triglycerides in the liver.

(d) **True**   This is another property of the isobutyric acid derivatives. In terms of side-effects they are similar although clofibrate however appears more likely to accelerate the development of gallstones. Incidentally all have an association with myalgias.

(e) **False**   As in (a).

---

287 (a) **False**   It is proportional to concentration gradient with a limiting effect because of the saturation of the carrier.

(b) **True**

(c) **False**   Tissue blood flow is the limiting factor.

(d) **True**

(e) **False**

288 (a) **True**

(b) **False**   It indicates the extent to which the drug reaches its site of action.

(c) **False**   It is between 10 and 30 per cent due to extensive first-pass metabolism.

(d) **False**   It is much lower.

(e) **True**

289 (a) **False**

(b) **False**   This drug is almost entirely restricted to the intravascular compartment and its volume of distribution is 4–5 litres in an average adult.

(c) **False**   Drugs which distribute extensively into tissues have very large volumes of distribution.

(d) **True**   In the blood or tissues.

(e) **True**

290 Protein binding:
   (a) Of basic drugs usually occurs to plasma albumin.
   (b) Of acidic drugs usually occurs to alpha-1-glycoprotein.
   (c) Changes are insignificant for drugs that are over 95 per cent protein bound.
   (d) Is of significance if a drug has a low therapeutic index.
   (e) Is of significance if a drug has a small volume of distribution.

291 In first order kinetics:
   (a) The elimination half-life increases with each additional dose of the drug.
   (b) The rate constant is expressed in ml/kg/hour.
   (c) The amount of drug excreted unchanged in the urine is proportional to the dose.
   (d) The plot of log concentration against time is a straight line.
   (e) The area under the log concentration–time graph is not proportional to the amount of drug administered.

292 The clearance of a drug:
   (a) Is the product of blood flow and extraction ratio.
   (b) Is dependent on the volume of distribution.
   (c) That has a low extraction ratio is largely independent of blood flow.
   (d) Varies with time in first order kinetics.
   (e) Through several organs can be summed by multiplying the individual organ clearances.

293 When drugs are administered by a continuous infusion:
   (a) The time to attain a steady state is independent of the rate of infusion.
   (b) Elimination half-life plays no part in attaining the steady state.
   (c) The rate at which a steady state concentration is attained is independent of the volume of distribution.
   (d) A loading dose equivalent to the product of volume of distribution and the target steady state concentration helps in attaining that concentration more rapidly.
   (e) The dose required to maintain a steady state is the sum of the concentration required and the rate of clearance.

290 (a) **False**   Generally acidic drugs such as warfarin or diazepam bind to albumin.

   (b) **False**   Usually basic drugs such as propranolol bind to it.

   (c) **False**   Changes in protein binding of such drugs are very significant.

   (d) **True**

   (e) **True**   It is a feature of highly-bound drugs. Phenytoin and theophylline are clinically important drugs, with the potential for adverse interactions on the basis of protein binding.

291 (a) **False**   It is constant until the time the kinetics become zero order.

   (b) **False**

   (c) **True**   If any was excreted!

   (d) **True**

   (e) **False**

292 (a) **True**

   (b) **False**   The elimination half-life, but not the clearance, changes by changes in the volume of distribution.

   (c) **True**

   (d) **False**   It is a constant.

   (e) **False**   They are just added.

293 (a) **True**

   (b) **False**   The steady state concentration is attained in about five half-lives, provided first order kinetics apply.

   (c) **True**

   (d) **True**

   (e) **False**   It is the product of the two.

294 The figure shows log-dose–response curves for two drugs where:

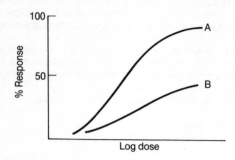

(a) Drug A shows affinity and high efficacy.
(b) Drug B shows less intrinsic activity than A.
(c) Drug B is actually drug A in the presence of a non-competitive antagonist.
(d) Drug B is actually drug A in the presence of a competitive antagonist.
(e) Drug B represents a non-competitive antagonist of drug A.

295 Metabolic processes:
(a) Of 'Phase I' are typified by conjugation.
(b) Of 'Phase II' are essentially synthetic in nature.
(c) Involving drugs generally results in more lipid-soluble compounds.
(d) Involving hydrolysis are mostly restricted to amides and esters.
(e) Involving mercapturic acid conjugation is inversely proportional to the glutathione concentration.

296 In statistics the term or concept of:
(a) A 'statistic' refers to populations.
(b) 'Precision' describes how close statistics are to each other.
(c) 'The central limit theorem' accounts for the significance of the normal distribution.
(d) 'Bias' is used to describe how far a parameter lies from a statistic.
(e) A 'parameter' refers to a constant.

294 (a) **True**   It is an agonist.
(b) **True**   It cannot produce the same maximum response as A.
(c) **False**   If this was the case then drug B would not have its dose–
response curve shifted so much to the right of A, rather it would
be in the same position as A but with a much smaller response
and a different slope.
(d) **False**   In this case B would ultimately attain the same maximum
response as A, by increasing the dose. The slope of the curves
would also be similar.
(e) **True**

295 (a) **False**   The Phase I reactions are oxidation, reduction or hydrolysis.
(b) **True**   Processes such as conjugation create glucuronide or acetyl
derivatives of the metabolites produced from Phase I reactions.
(c) **False**   The ultimate aim of metabolic processes is to produce water-
soluble products that can be eliminated.
(d) **True**
(e) **False**   It is directly related. Mercapturic acid conjugates are used by
the body to deal with the intermediates formed by drugs like paracetamol with glutathione. Thus depletion of glutathione results in
accumulation of toxic intermediate metabolites.

296 (a) **False**   A statistic is a numerical value summarizing sample data; as
such it does not refer to a population but a sample of that
population.
(b) **True**
(c) **True**   If sets of observations come from a normal distribution then the
mean of each set of observations will approach the mean of the
normal distribution as the number of observations increases.
(d) **True**
(e) **True**   Since it is based on all the subjects in the actual population as
distinct from a sample it will not show sampling error! In inferential statistics people are seeking to describe the parameters of
a population from the statistics of a sample.

297 In statistical terms in groups of 100 subjects:
  (a) 97 per cent of subjects will be within the height range of 105–135 cm if the mean of the group is 120 cm and the standard deviation 10 cm.
  (b) 99 per cent of subjects will have their systolic arterial pressure within the range 90–110 mm Hg if the mean systolic pressure of the group is 100 mm Hg, with a standard error of the mean of 10 mm Hg.
  (c) The results are clinically significant between two groups if the P value is less than 5 per cent.
  (d) The P value quantifies the probability of making a type II error.
  (e) Student's t test is appropriate for testing the significance of the difference between two groups of observations.

298 In a study of 100 patients it was found that obesity and the incidence of coronary artery narrowing had a positive correlation coefficient of 0.6 and the correlation coefficient between coronary artery narrowing and high-density lipoprotein levels was 0.001. Therefore:
  (a) Obesity is a cause of coronary artery narrowing.
  (b) Pearsons correlation coefficient would be an appropriate measure of the correlation between the coronary artery narrowing and obesity.
  (c) Spearman's correlation coefficient could be used to measure the association between high-density-lipoprotein levels and coronary artery narrowing.
  (d) As obesity increases there is a tendency for coronary artery narrowing to increase.
  (e) There is no linear relationship between levels of high-density lipoproteins and coronary narrowing.

299 In naming scales or variables:
  (a) Gender is on a nominal scale.
  (b) Your examination number is on a nominal scale.
  (c) Temperature in °F is on an interval scale.
  (d) Time is on a ratio scale.
  (e) Dependent variables are so-called because they depend on the experimenter choosing them.

297 (a) **False**   As a rule of thumb one should expect 95 per cent of observations to be within two standard deviations (SD) on either side of the mean provided the distribution of results is approximately normal. The 'normal distribution' (which has a precise mathematical definition) is represented by a symmetrical bell-shaped curve with two points of inflection. It started off as a way of describing games of chance but was subsequently used in biology by Adolph Quetelet (1796–1855) who found that the heights of French soldiers were approximately normally distributed, from which he deduced that the mean of the distribution was nature's 'ideal' so that the observations on either side of the mean represented an 'error'. Hence the use of this term in referring to deviations from the mean.

  (b) **False**   The 'standard error of the mean' (SEM) is quoted here. Authors sometimes quote this because it is smaller than the standard deviation but it does not immediately provide information about the distribution of results, the relationship is SD equals SEM multiplied by the square root of the sample size. As a rule of thumb there is a roughly a 95 per cent chance that the true mean of the **population** from which the sample is drawn lies within two standard errors of the mean of the **sample** mean.

  (c) **False**   P value is indicative of statistical significance of the results and not the clinical significance.

  (d) **False**   It provides no information about this, it tells us the probability of not rejecting the null hypothesis when it is false.

  (e) **True**   Provided that the data conforms to a normal distribution and we are only testing between **two** groups only.

298 (a) **False**   No causal relationship is established, although the two may be present together.

  (b) **True**   Provided the data follow a normal or approximately normal distribution.

  (c) **True**   This makes no assumptions of normality, and so can be used with a subjective ranking of coronary artery narrowing. It is very similar mathematically to Pearsons correlation coefficient but is less sensitive.

  (d) **True**

  (e) **True**   Just because the correlation is near zero does not mean that no relationship exists.

299 (a) **True**   When using words although often for the purposes of calculations male and female will be given code numbers. These numbers bear no meaningful relationship to each other, they are just tags.

  (b) **True**   It does not rank the holder in position in the class.

  (c) **True**   A given difference has the same meaning anywhere along the scale, but the zero point of the scale is arbitrary.

  (d) **True**   Because now ratios have meanings e.g. 2 minutes is twice as long as one minute.

  (e) **False**   This is a description of the independent variable, the dependent variable constitutes the data the experimenter collects.

300 The chi-square test:
  (a) Is a descriptive statistic.
  (b) Is often used to analyse categorical data.
  (c) Yields a value that is greater the larger the number of subjects.
  (d) Cannot be used on percentages.
  (e) Cannot be used if more than 20 per cent of the cells have an expected frequency of less than five.

300 (a) **False** Descriptive statistics are such things as the standard deviation, percentile rank etc.; their purpose is to describe the data. An inferential statistic is used to say something about a population.

(b) **True** Categorical data is also known as frequency data or qualitative data like taste preference as distinct from quantitative data such as a subject's weight.

(c) **False** The value is greater not when the number of subjects is large but either when a greater number of categories are being tested or when the differences being tested are large.

(d) **True** These need to be changed to frequencies.

(e) **True** The test is not appropriate if the expected frequency in a number of cells is very small (because the test assumes that if the experiment in question was repeated many times the frequencies in a cell would be normally distributed about the expected frequency).

Recommended Reading

Bowman WC, Rand MJ: *Textbook Of Pharmacology*. Blackwell Scientific Publications: Oxford, 1980.

Craig CR, Stitzel RE: *Modern Pharmacology*. Little, Brown and Company: Boston, 1990.

Dundee JW, Clarke RSJ, McCaughey W: *Clinical Anaesthetic Pharmacology*. Churchill Livingstone: London, 1991.

Feely J (Ed): *New Drugs*. British Medical Journal: London, 1991.

Gilles HC, Rogers HJ, Spector RG, Trounce JR: *A Textbook Of Clinical Pharmacology*. Edward Arnold: London, 1989.

Goodman AG, Rall TW, Nies AS, Taylor P: *Goodman and Gilman's The Pharmacological Basis Of Therapeutics*. Pergamon Press: Oxford, 1990.

Opie LH (Ed): *Drugs For The Heart*. Grune and Stratton: Orlando, 1987.

Wood M, Wood AJJ: *Drugs And Anesthesia*. Williams and Wilkins: Baltimore, 1990.